The Nursing Home Guide

The NURSING HOME Guide

A Doctor Reveals
What You Need to Know
About Long-Term Care

JOSHUA D. SCHOR, M.D.

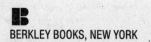

BERKLEY BOOKS, NEW YORK

THE BERKLEY PUBLISHING GROUP
Published by the Penguin Group
Penguin Group (USA) Inc.
375 Hudson Street, New York, New York 10014, USA
Penguin Group (Canada), 90 Eglinton Avenue East, Suite 700, Toronto, Ontario M4P 2Y3, Canada
(a division of Pearson Penguin Canada Inc.)
Penguin Books Ltd., 80 Strand, London WC2R 0RL, England
Penguin Group Ireland, 25 St. Stephen's Green, Dublin 2, Ireland (a division of Penguin Books Ltd.)
Penguin Group (Australia), 250 Camberwell Road, Camberwell, Victoria 3124, Australia
(a division of Pearson Australia Group Pty. Ltd.)
Penguin Books India Pvt. Ltd., 11 Community Centre, Panchsheel Park, New Delhi—110 017, India
Penguin Group (NZ), 67 Apollo Drive, Rosedale, North Shore 0632, New Zealand
(a division of Pearson New Zealand Ltd.)
Penguin Books (South Africa) (Pty.) Ltd., 24 Sturdee Avenue, Rosebank, Johannesburg 2196,
South Africa

Penguin Books Ltd., Registered Offices: 80 Strand, London WC2R 0RL, England

This book is an original publication of The Berkley Publishing Group.

PUBLISHER'S NOTE: Every effort has been made to ensure that the information contained in this book is complete and accurate. While the author has disguised the identities of some persons portrayed, the work is a factual report. However, neither the publisher nor the author is engaged in rendering professional advice or services to the individual reader. The ideas, procedures, and suggestions contained in this book are not intended as a substitute for consulting with your physician. All matters regarding your health require medical supervision. Neither the author nor the publisher shall be liable or responsible for any loss or damage allegedly arising from any information or suggestion in this book.

While the author has made every effort to provide accurate telephone numbers and Internet addresses at the time of publication, neither the publisher nor the author assumes any responsibility for errors, or for changes that occur after publication. Further, publisher does not have any control over and does not assume any responsibility for author or third-party websites or their content.

PRINTING HISTORY
Berkley trade paperback edition / December 2008

Library of Congress Cataloging-in-Publication Data

Schor, Joshua D.
    The nursing home guide : a doctor reveals what you need to know about long-term care / Joshua D. Schor.
      p. cm.
    ISBN 978-0-425-22378-9
    1. Nursing homes. I. Title.

    RA997.S366 2008
    362.16—dc22

                                                                    2008035654

PRINTED IN THE UNITED STATES OF AMERICA

10 9 8 7 6 5 4 3 2 1

Most Berkley Books are available at special quantity discounts for bulk purchases for sales, promotions, premiums, fund-raising, or educational use. Special books, or book excerpts, can also be created to fit specific needs.

For details, write: Special Markets, The Berkley Publishing Group, 375 Hudson Street, New York, New York 10014.

For Lori...Some luck lies...

Acknowledgments

In writing this book, I hope I have spoken for the many patients and their families I have come to know. It is to them that I owe sincere thanks. For those who I have not met, I hope this book can be a useful guide. My agent, Susan Cohen, has been patient and encouraging. Seeing her and her son, Julian, is always a special treat. My editor, Denise Silvestro, is an expert at her craft, and only because she is so tactful and genuine was I able to restrain myself and write more guide than memoir. I also thank Denise's assistant, Meredith Giordan, who has been especially helpful.

I have had wonderful colleagues and friends in the long-term care world: first and foremost those on the staff of my own home away from home, Daughters of Israel in West Orange, New Jersey. Larry Gelfand has always been a supportive, warm, and wise director and in no small way inspired me to commit my thoughts to paper. Mary Spielvogel has been the biggest-hearted director of nursing and has earned a good retirement. Both Susan Grosser and Susan Harris are carrying on the challenge and are models of hard work, intelligence, and grace. In no particular order, I owe great thanks to Adena Twersky, Lisa Verdon, Muriel Bradshaw, Chris Mooney, Sandy Shore, Tom Tierney, Barbara Quinlan, Colleen Thompson, Rabbi Zvi Karpel, Barbara London, Pat Watson, Lydia Stanislaus, Dawn Thompson, Argenett Anderson, Sharon Glaser, Eve Goldberg, Li Schuman, Karen Callahan, Jennifer Rutberg, Joann Digiovanni, Mark Sapoznick, Sylvia Goodman, Joyce Silverman, Sophia McGhee, Anne Berry, Steven Finkler, Gary Beinhacker, Jan Ball, and the Daughters of Israel Board of Governors.

My chief mentors in geriatrics, Drs. Lewis Lipsitz, Kenneth Minaker, and Ed Kaminskas, were unstinting in their time and infallible in their advice. Dr. Phil McCarthy was the most inspiring and dedicated resident a medical student could wish for. My colleagues at Evercare have taught me how to put good care and good ideas into good practice; their nurse practitioners and clinical service managers are transforming the face of long-term care.

With great family, I have been greatly rewarded. My parents, Joe and Sandy, took wonderful care of their parents and my extended sibling clan, Starry, Walter, Gideon, Beth, Freddie, and Marcie Lee, have done nothing less with ours. Thanks to Rita and Laura for love and support. If a book on nursing homes could have a muse, it is surely my wife, Lori. She has a sensitive ear and a charitable and loving soul. With each successive birth of our three daughters, Lori and I recognized that we were increasingly blessed. Noemi, Shayna, and Rafaella: Thank you for lots of love and loads of laughs, but do what you have to do. Mom and I will be proud to be your parents in whatever nursing home you choose for us. But choose well!

Contents

Introduction

Several years ago, I read a newspaper story that has stuck with me. It concerned an elderly Arizona gentleman who had been a felon for much of his life. For some years he had gone straight, but owing to desperate finances, very bad health, and perhaps an unflagging criminal bent, he held up a convenience store from his wheelchair at age ninety-two. His getaway was none too swift and as he exited the wheelchair ramp the police apprehended him. He was soon convicted and a wise judge deliberated on the sentence. The judge observed that the man was not a flight risk and that he badly needed care. The judge offered him a choice between seven to ten years in prison or admission to a local nursing home. The felon responded that he'd rather take his chances in prison because he'd never get out of a nursing home alive.

We have probably all thought about having to put a parent, an uncle, an aunt, or someone dear to us in a nursing home—and like the felon, would prefer just about any other option. For instance, what about assisted living or foster care for seniors? I will explore those, too, but what if you conclude that a nursing home *is* necessary? Some of us have promised (as have I and my siblings) *not* to put a father or mother in a nursing home. These promises are often made toward the end of a holiday meal like Thanksgiving. After everyone has finished the main course, sipped plenty of wine, and dessert is about to begin, the topic arises. It is usually one of the elders in our midst: "Do you remember Aunt Gussie? Her son Irving just put her in a nursing home." Silence, and then the other shoe drops. "Promise me, you'll never stick me in some godforsaken place like that." Another pregnant pause and then, "Sure, Mom. Pass the rice pudding."

As a geriatrician in the practice of long-term care, I've heard this story a hundred times. Because I specialize in this field, I know that almost everyone sees long-term care as a last resort. Many of us have made promises that we cannot keep. It can break our hearts to have to put someone we love and who more than likely raised us and sacrificed for us into a nursing home.

So what's a child to do? Is a good nursing home really that hard to find? This book will help guide you in your search for a good home. And it will help you make the most of that home *after* your loved one has moved in. I will try to paint an accurate picture of the state of long-term care and how to be sure the resident of the home gets the best treatment available.

The cast of characters on a nursing home staff is large and deserves discussion, too. You have limited amounts of time, and being a caring and devoted family member or friend will require time to visit, to call, and to advocate for your loved one. I hope to help you understand who is who in a nursing home so you can avoid the "runaround" and instead share time with your loved one.

I have learned to place myself in the shoes of my patients whenever I can. One of my most memorable was a gentleman named Harry who was 104 when we first met. He had been a tailor and still threaded a needle with ease. I had just been introduced as the new doctor on the unit. He recently had prostate problems and had been to a urologist (a *man's* best friend, my cousin the urologist tells me) who had ordered some lab tests. Sensing he might get more information from me than from the last doctor, he swept up to me like a middle linebacker. I checked with the lab and was told that the results were not ready. I told Harry there was nothing to report but every half hour he approached me while I was working to ask again. I then made the mistake of saying something like, "Harry, what's the rush? You've lived one hundred and four years. What difference would a day or two make?" Harry grabbed me by the lapel of my bright white lab coat and said, "Doc, you don't understand. I'm one hundred and four. Every minute counts."

I adore my work. I've done many other things in medicine, from working in emergency rooms to reviewing insurance applications, but I've never done anything as fulfilling as the work I perform as medical director of a three-hundred-bed nursing home. I tell the students who work with me that long-term care is an acquired taste; they quickly understand what I mean. It's *not* for everyone. But then many of you never thought you'd need to read a book like this. We make the best of the situation in which we find ourselves.

I'm anxious to tell the good, the bad, and the ugly. And I hope you'll come to see that it is *not* all ugly out there. I've witnessed some moving and beautiful moments in my work and I hope to share these with you, too. I admire many of my medical colleagues. Great doctors have inspired me and I carry their stories and wisdom and bits of their bedside manner with me every day. However, I can't help but see some of my colleagues' failings, too. My aim is not to be harsh but to be helpful and if I appear to go overboard at times, I take responsibility and apologize,

There's plenty of good to be said about nursing homes. As

a society, we're quick to blame external factors when things go wrong. But sometimes stuff just happens: People age, the good times end, and friends abandon friends. The comedian Robert Klein has a routine on aging and what a bust Florida is. I paraphrase, "What's so great about Florida for the elderly? I took my parents down there. They were sixty-five...great health...played cards. Now I have to bring them up north again thirty years later. And look at them, old, wrinkled, like ghosts! What the hell good did Florida do for them anyway?" Too often we expect miracles and are disappointed.

We all have the opportunity in life to learn more and do better, but sometimes we miss the chance. Please consider this an offering to help you not miss that chance. Even if you couldn't keep your promise—Thanksgiving dinner or not—let's make the most of what lies ahead.

The chapters in this book represent key currents that run through long-term care and geriatrics. If you are looking for a topic that is not listed as a chapter heading, consult the index. For example, I address bedsores (now known as pressure ulcers) in many different chapters depending on the context rather than as its own topic.

I have changed the names of all patients that appear in this book, but all of the stories are true. It is my hope that they will help you with whatever decisions you may have to make. I have also referred to websites that might be useful.

Historically Speaking:
A Brief History of
Long-Term Care

For those of you who love a good meal but prefer to savor some appetizers first, I offer this section as a historical introduction. I realize that you may have pressing concerns and need the lowdown in a hurry. If so, then by all means skip right to the entrée by beginning at chapter 1. When you get a chance, though, think about returning and reading this at your leisure. The history of the nursing home reform movement is absorbing. It will help you understand the ins and outs of present-day nursing homes and how to get the most out of what lies ahead.

Early History

Nursing homes are almost entirely a product of the twentieth century. What few long-term institutions existed before then were "warehouses" for the insane or the criminally insane. I love anything that Mozart composed and *Amadeus* is one of my favorite movies. A memorable flashback scene takes place near the beginning of the film. Antonio Salieri, Mozart's great rival, looks back to his own youth and his intense competition with Mozart. The viewer is brought in to "see" Salieri by passing through filthy halls filled with grotesque lunatics, many of whom are chained to walls. As we hear their crazy and demented riffs, it becomes clear that we are in a version of Bedlam, the venerable insane asylum of eighteenth-century London. This model evolved over centuries to become a kind of psychiatric *hospital* with wards, rooms, corridors, and staff grouped centrally at a *station*. For want of a better model, many nursing homes still reflect this structure. The best nursing homes today look more like "homes" than asylums or hospitals, but the "medical" model still predominates. The good homes have incorporated features of a "rest home" or "retirement home" with easy chairs, living rooms, and fireplaces, but one still finds medical charts, medication carts, call bells, and paging systems.

Today there is a growing movement known as "culture change" exemplified by such programs as the Eden Alternative and the Pioneer Network. Homes that subscribe to these models rid themselves, as much as they can, of hospital appearances. Some have pet cats and dogs running freely, spacious outdoor areas to roam (even if video-monitored), and smaller kitchens rather than communal dining halls. Some new homes were designed with this in mind and if you're lucky enough to live near one, it behooves you to take a look when picking a home. Then again, if your family member or you hate pets, it's likely not the place for either of you.

As homes evolved in this country, there needed to be someone to pay the bill. Until the 1930s this someone was either the individual who needed to be in the nursing home or her family. With the passage of FDR's Social Security Act in 1935, public funds became available to pay for some types of long-term care. The quantum leap forward occurred when Lyndon Johnson forged Medicare and Medicaid as part of his Great Society in the 1960s. While not created with long-term care in mind, the two federal health programs now pay for the majority of long-term care in this country. Medicare and Medicaid are administered by CMS, Centers for Medicare & Medicaid Services (formerly HCFA, the Health Care Financing Administration). It is an open question as to how or even whether the state and federal governments will continue to pay for long-term care; no one envisioned these programs paying for it in the first place.

Bergman and Hess: *The Times* to the Rescue

Since the government was increasingly paying for nursing home care, it gradually became interested in the quality of care. States performed annual inspections or "surveys," but conditions in many homes were problematic. That is, at least, until *The New York Times* seized on the issue in the early 1970s. *The Times* published a series of detailed articles that in fine journalistic fashion exposed a large nursing home for what it was: a warehouse for the elderly not dissimilar to the asylum in *Amadeus*. The effect of these articles was seismic.

The reporter credited with blowing the lid off the nursing home industry is John L. Hess. Hess wrote notably about the Towers Nursing Home in New York City on West 106th Street, which at the time was owned by Bernard Bergman. Mr. Bergman had a history of deplorable practices in his nursing home empire. At the peak of his career, he or his family had significant financial stakes in close to one hundred homes in and out of New York. He was an ordained orthodox rabbi who was a contributor to the Nixon reelection effort and once gave the opening prayer in the House of Representatives. He was born in Hungary and came from a family with a pedigree of crime. His mother and stepfather had been caught smuggling large amounts of heroin hidden inside prayer books out of Europe.

Hess uncovered irregularities in Bergman's billing practices, such as continuing to bill Medicaid for a resident who had died almost a year prior. Bergman was investigated and prosecuted by a young New York politician named Andrew Stein, who even uncovered a connection with the Mafia. Stein, with Hess, exposed a veritable web of nursing home crimes.

Equally as shocking as the financial fraud was the terrible care that was witnessed in the Towers home and in many other homes. To demonstrate how widespread the problem was, when the Towers Nursing Home "voluntarily" suspended operations in December 1974, of the thirty-one nursing homes to which residents were transferred, eight were themselves labeled "unsatisfactory" by the department of health. Reporters who entered these homes witnessed unclean conditions and inattentive staff. They also observed streams of elderly residents arranged in wheelchairs with little purpose and nothing to do. Many were fastened to their chairs by restraints and appeared to be struggling to get out. Others seemed drugged (*chemically restrained* in the jargon) as they leaned helplessly to one side, drooling and mumbling incoherently. For the most part, the nursing home staff ignored the reporters, and the administrators were unresponsive to their requests for interviews.

These articles appeared on the heels of the exposé of the Willowbrook State School in 1972 (a "school" for the mentally retarded in New York City with deplorable conditions) and were more bad news for the most vulnerable in our society. While the Willowbrook saga was sobering and even shocking, it did not strike the universal chord that the articles on the Towers Nursing Home did. Readers of the articles identified on a very personal level. Who did not have a beloved parent, or an aunt or uncle, that lived in a nursing home? Many a reader even projected that he or she might need to stay in a home someday. People were not afraid of becoming "retarded" but they were afraid of becoming old. The outrage was deep and pervasive.

The federal government convicted Bernard Bergman and sentenced him to four months in prison for Medicaid fraud. He was also sentenced to one year in prison by New York State and paid millions of dollars in fines. Bergman was referred to as the "meanest man in New York" at a time when that sobriquet was hardwon, but the Bergman scandal arguably did more to improve the care of the elderly in long-term facilities than any other event.

The movement for reform gathered steam and landed in the laps of Washington legislators. The extent of the abuses outraged and embarrassed them into action. Hearing after hearing documented the poor care in nursing homes, and advocacy groups such as the Gray Panthers maintained pressure on HCFA to do something. There were also financial pressures, since Uncle Sam was footing a growing portion of the bill. Citizens and congressional figures demanded action.

By the early 1980s, HCFA assigned the problem to a highly regarded think tank known as the Institute of Medicine. Its charge became improving the quality of care in nursing homes quickly and decisively. The institute in turn contracted with a number of academic groups (mainly Brown University) and arrived at several mechanisms to bring about change.

Reform

The major finding of the Institute of Medicine and its subcontractors was that nursing homes did not appreciate residents as individuals but rather treated them as amorphous and homogeneous gray-haired boarders. The key to change was to *individualize* the care. The staff at each home had to understand that each resident was unique and deserved his or her own plan of care.

The long-term care industry has spent the last twenty years ferreting out ways to achieve this end. Education has a parallel in what is known as "differentiated learning." The principle is the same: no more "one size fits all" approach whether it's for first graders in primary school or "last graders" in nursing homes. While local school boards can expand budgets, nursing homes cannot. Increased staff time required more dollars and the government demanded that the homes foot most of the bill. What HCFA and the Institute of Medicine wanted, though, was for the homes to be creative and work *smarter*, not *harder*.

The reform movement crystallized in the Nursing Home Reform Act, which was part of "OBRA 87." OBRA stands for Omnibus Budget Reconciliation Act and goes by that moniker because the budget process for 1987 included long-term care funding. OBRA tackled several issues and chief among them was the creation of a lengthy assessment tool called the Minimum Data Set or MDS. The need for the MDS spoke volumes about nursing homes. First, it suggested that the industry did not possess even the most basic mechanisms to understand and recognize who its own residents were and what made them tick. Second, "the feds" did not trust the homes to arrive at or create those tools on their own.

In other words, the jig was up. The gravy train had run its last route. The days of billing—or, in cases like Bergman's, *over*billing—HCFA for every resident day without regard to quality were gone. HCFA mandated that the staff of a home complete an assessment on every resident at the time of admission, and every quarter thereafter. HCFA also required an MDS assessment whenever there was a major change in status of a resident, such as a stroke or a fracture.

If ever there is a mixed blessing, it is the MDS...and "minimum," my derrière. It carries such a profusion of information that it makes Bill Gates's tax form look like a parking ticket. The MDS analyzes each resident across eighteen fields or domains stretching from skin care to health status to spiritual and emotional states. To that end, as long as the staff is reasonably well trained, it succeeds nicely. The rub has always been that the forms take so much time to complete, it diminishes staff time that could better be spent with the residents.

There have been several more iterations of the MDS since its inception. Because of the nature of the MDS, and how many aspects of the residents' lives are involved, it is desirable to have all disciplines participate in completing it. At our home, the nurses, social workers, activity therapists, physical and occupational therapists, and dieticians meet regularly to complete the forms. The certified nursing assistants and orderlies know more about the residents' day-to-day needs than anyone. They do not always participate in the exercise but the head nurse obtains their input beforehand.

The average team at our home spends about a day a week completing the MDS forms just to cover its fifty residents. I see them huddled around a computer (the MDS is all electronic now) for hours on end. Shouldn't they be at the bedside of patients? Since the government does not trust the industry, the question is moot. The MDS *must* be done. One wonders if one hundred years from now, a nursing home administrator will extract from a time capsule a crumpled MDS form and try to understand how it might have changed an industry. While the jury may be out, the MDS is here to stay.

If the MDS is completed and launched into cyberspace, this alone achieves little. The designers of the MDS made sure that the findings would translate into real changes for the residents. For example, the MDS might reveal that in the psychological domain the resident has been crying every afternoon. The MDS then triggers a series of prompts to help identify the problem. These suggestions collectively comprise the RAP or resident assessment protocol. Has the resident recently lost a family member? Does the resident have a prior history of depression? Is the resident participating in activities as she had before or is she becoming a loner and isolating herself in her room? The obvious suggestion would be to increase as many social contacts as possible and get in touch with the family. In addition, the team would more than likely notify the physician and ask if psychiatric or psychological evaluation is warranted. Thus the data from the MDS does not sit in a clinical vacuum but solicits interventions to help the resident.

If one stands back and takes a dispassionate view, the MDS is a terrific success. It has resulted in more specific and appropriate care for the almost two million residents of long-term care in this country. It has forced all the players on the long-term care team to be accountable, responsible, and even creative in solving problems. It has answered the government's demand to achieve the "highest practicable" quality of care for the residents.

There is also no escaping how time-consuming it is. Some homes undermine the system by hiring a full-time "MDS coordinator" nurse to do the paperwork. This practice is perfectly legal but in my mind it violates the spirit of the MDS, which was to leverage the primary staff's daily interactions with the residents.

The MDS is an industry unto itself and I will discuss later in this book how surveyors use the data to review a home. Reimbursement from the feds may be keyed off the MDS in the future and in some states that future is now. To get bogged down here in the minutiae of the MDS would be to delay the goal of familiarizing you with how to choose a home and understanding the culture of long-term care. Suffice it to say that the creation of the MDS was a quantum leap forward in the quality of most homes. One could argue that federal and state agencies more closely monitor and regulate nursing homes than any other facet of the health care industry.

How exactly do we find the best home? The first four chapters of this book focus on choosing the right home, while the next eight chapters concentrate on moving into and living in the home and how to make the most of it for your loved one. I hope these insights inform and guide you, and help you make the most of one of the toughest decisions you may ever have to face.

Part I

Finding the Right Home

1

Choosing a Home

Sub-Acute vs. Long-Term Care

There are two different scenarios that may require you to consider a nursing home. One depends on a situation of *urgency* or *crisis* and the other on answering the question: *Has the time finally arrived?*

It is easier in a sense to consider the crisis situation first. If you're reading this book in a hurry, leafing through to get some quick answers, my guess is that this scenario involves you. Most often the urgency is based on your family member having been admitted to the hospital for any of a number of reasons and discharge back to home is not feasible.

The other scenario—in which a family feels the time has arrived and it is no longer safe at home—has become far less the norm. In our own nursing home, I would have to think to recall the last person who was admitted from home rather than a hospital or another nursing facility. With home care, day care, assisted living (see end of this chapter), and the like, there is a plethora of ways to keep someone out of a nursing home. Almost routinely now, it is a fall, a fracture, a stroke, or some other serious medical situation that signifies a change drastic enough to require a more supervised environment. Crisis or not, what follows will serve as a road map to choosing a good home.

Back in the day, hospitals were able to keep patients for weeks, even months, at a time. When a fifty-year-old man suffered a heart attack, the standard treatment was bed rest for several weeks in the hospital. Therapists would eventually begin a slow program to get the man on his feet and discharge him home. An eighty-five-year-old woman who fell and fractured a hip had surgery quickly and remained in the acute hospital for weeks to receive training on how to walk again. When she was independent, she went home. This was a great business for the hospital. It charged the insurance company for every day and was paid top dollar for it. Things began to change in the early 1980s when costs escalated quickly and the insurance companies placed limits on what they would pay. A suddenly beleaguered hospital system needed to adapt to a brave new world.

The coup de grâce occurred when Medicare, by far the biggest insurer in the nation, announced similar limitations in the early 1980s. Now instead of paying for each day, each lab test, and each hour of therapy, there was a fixed amount it would pay for each stay. For the elderly woman with a hip fracture, it no longer mattered whether she was hospitalized for two days or for two weeks, Medicare would pay only one fixed amount for the entire stay (known as a DRG or diagnosis related group).

This turned hospital practice on its head. The incentive switched from long, plodding admissions to the hospital needing to get the patient out as soon as possible. The goal was how to "turn over" the bed.

You may or may not have heard of "length of stay," but it has become the bane of many physicians' existence. Length of stay is literally how long a patient remains in the hospital as measured against the ideal stays determined by the new DRG payment system. An extended length of stay means the hospital is losing money. Given the parameters of the new system, one can hardly blame the hospitals for seeming to rush patients out. These constraints have driven many fine (and some not so fine) institutions into bankruptcy and many of the remainder are barely breaking even.

Understanding this dynamic is crucial because it has spawned a new layer of staff in the hospital known alternatively as "discharge planners" or "case managers." These supervisors substitute for what social workers traditionally did in the hospital (and some still do). Whereas social workers cared a lot about the well-being and emotional stability of a patient and that the discharge plan would work, the discharge planners are leaner and meaner. I certainly don't want to imply that they do not care. Many of those with whom I've worked are caring and responsible professionals. But they are hired to do a job that can run counter to what is best for the patient.

From the moment one is admitted to the hospital, the planner is already designing a plan for discharge. This is not wholly bad. Hospitals, it has been said, are no places for sick people. They are noisy and cold and not conducive to rest. They are filled with terribly resistant bacteria—a problem that is only getting worse. Most alarming, errors and iatrogenesis (when doctors cause bad things to happen to good patients) are rampant.

So as soon as the medical team and nurses feel the patient is ready to go, it is best they plan accordingly. Sometimes things get rushed, and I've certainly felt the pressure to discharge someone before he or she was ready. Many doctors are more conservative in their practice and keep patients in the hospital much longer than is needed. The challenge, as with anything, is striking the right balance.

Question Authority

When the discharge planner tells you that your family member is ready for discharge, ask a few pointed questions.

- *Is the physician in complete agreement with discharge?* If so, it is almost always worth hearing this *from* the physician and it is reasonable to wait for a callback from the doctor to confirm.

- *If the plan is for discharge home, is this a safe plan?* In other words, is the planner aware of the home environment—with steps, rugs, stoops, etc.—and has he or she taken this into account.

- *Do the therapists think the patient can negotiate this and if help is needed, have arrangements been made?* It is your right to ask if a home evaluation can be done since you have valid safety concerns. Some hospitals can provide this service but more often they will send the visiting nurse association (VNA) that will be providing help anyway.

- *Are there any wounds that need dressing and if so how often, by whom, and who will follow up?* Medicare and most insurance companies will pay for a limited amount of home care for a period of weeks following the hospitalization. Have the correct referrals with a home health agency (and VNA) been made?

- *Is the medical treatment completed or will it be completed after discharge?* When you visit your family member on the day of discharge, see if she is still tethered to an oxygen tube or an IV cord or urinary catheter. This is a very common mistake on discharge and you must insist that all such appliances be removed unless needed. The hospital's failure to think about this represents poor care and may well be the physician's responsibility. Often the physician will simply not remember or be so oblivious that he/she forgets that the patient will be going into the real world again and not nestled in the cocoon of the hospital.

It is perfectly valid to refuse discharge and raise Cain if no one has answers to these questions. Most hospitals have patient advocates or "patient reps" for just these problems and they should be brought in if you receive any flack or rolling of the eyes. My mother, who at the time was receiving chemotherapy for advanced breast cancer, was once discharged with a needle literally sticking out of her chest from a "porta-cath" device. It fell upon me after I realized it just after a family dinner to remove it. Had I not been "in the know" it would have required a trip back to the ER with its attendant long wait. Worse yet, it might have become the source of an infection due to her weakened immune system. By no means do I wish to condemn outright a system that in many cases provides wonderful care. The period surrounding discharge is fraught, however, with many potential problems and it is worth slowing down to make sure your questions are answered.

Now we come to the major question: *If discharge to home is not feasible, what are the alternatives?* One certainly wants to know who is making the recommendation. A skilled case manager may be the one and that could be fine. While the physician may not be in the loop, it may be worth contacting him or her to understand what led to the recommendation. Often it is a clear-cut decision. If your family member is suffering from a disease such as osteomyelitis (infection of the bone) or endocarditis (infection of a heart valve) or even a severe pneumonia, she may need a prolonged course of antibiotics. This is often done via a special IV catheter (intravenous tube) known as a PICC line (peripherally inserted central catheter). With someone who is alert and spry, these kinds of treatments can be done at home, but in an older and frailer patient they are often best done at a nursing home.

In a case where a patient has suffered a broken hip or shoulder and cannot function at his or her prior level of independence, a stay at a rehabilitation center or nursing home is often advisable. The discharge planner *can* arrange nursing services and therapy at home, but it will be less intense and the therapist will visit less often.

A stroke will frequently result in the call for a rehab stay. It may necessitate these three major forms of therapy.

- *Physical therapy* to help with walking and changing positions

- *Occupational therapy* to assist in use of the arms and to help regain the so-called ADLs (activities of daily living, such as bathing, dressing, eating, moving from place to place, toileting, etc.)

- *Speech therapy* if speech, use of language, and/or swallowing was damaged by the stroke

Even if the patient was simply weakened by being in bed for a week or was recovering from a heart attack or congestive heart failure, he would probably qualify for a rehab stay.

Sub-Acute Care

Now let's define some terms. When we speak of a rehab stay we're talking about sub-acute care, Medicare Part A, or skilled nursing. Whatever the case manager or discharge planner calls it, the idea is to help a patient regain the function that was damaged due to the illness and hospital stay. Do you remember the DRGs and length of stay? These issues spawned a sub-acute care industry that really didn't exist prior to the 1980s. Sub-acute care is a Medicare benefit that pays, after a deductible, for 100% of the sub-acute rehab stay for the first twenty days and then 80% for days twenty through one hundred. Some Medigap or supplemental policies pay for the remainder. Many private insurance plans cover similar benefits though often not as generously as Medicare.

One can qualify through Medicare (and most private insurance plans) for sub-acute care with an appropriate diagnosis and two requirements: a three-night stay in the acute care hospital, and the ability to make gains in therapy. If a patient has significant dementia or utterly lacks the energy or motivation to cooperate, the therapists may need to terminate the therapy—and with that, the benefits from Medicare. Families appreciate sub-acute care because it is the one case in which Medicare pays for long-term care including room and board.

There are movements afoot to remove the three-day hospital requirement. The reason for this speaks to another large group that receives sub-acute care: those who are already admitted under long-term care. Let's say your family member has been admitted to a nursing home for increasing frailty due to arthritis, congestive heart failure, and mild dementia. After being there for quite some time, she falls and breaks a hip. Her physician admits her to the local hospital. After surgery to pin the hip and three more days to recover, she returns to the same nursing home. If that nursing home is licensed by Medicare for sub-acute care, she would qualify for the stay at Medicare's expense for twenty to one hundred days just as if her goal was to return to her own home. If the home does not provide sub-acute care, she may need a short stay at a home that does and then return to home base. She would, of course, need to meet the same requirements, which include the minimum three-day stay and the ability to cooperate and progress with a therapy plan of care.

That's beginning to be the dilemma. Medicare has figured out what all nursing homes have known for a long time. The more residents the home has on sub-acute care, the better will be their reimbursement by Medicare. It may not sound like a lot, but multiplied by several residents by many days by many years, it adds up to real money. Some nursing homes have been known to play the game of hospitalizing residents who perhaps could be treated for their ailment (pneumonia, for example) just as well at the nursing home. Of course this is a judgment call and not all hospital admissions can be prevented. Just as the homes make out, the physicians can also make out by having a larger census of hospitalized patients for which they can bill. So the incentives are all a bit screwy and weighted to sending someone to the hospital. The better-quality homes resist the urge and Medicare would love to avoid having to pay the much larger bill of a hospital stay, often running $12,000 to $15,000 or more. CMS (Centers for Medicare & Medicaid Services) is rumored to be contemplating rescinding the three-day requirement because in the end it will be cheaper for them to pay for ten or twenty days of appropriate rehab than to foot the bill for the hospital stay and *then* pay for the rehab anyway.

So stay tuned. Many geriatricians and long-term care organizations such as the American Medical Directors Association (AMDA) favor the change. Some innovative Medicare Advantage plans like Evercare (part of United HealthCare) have led the way and eliminated the three-day requirement for their insured residents. I think it would be a classic "win-win" since we could avoid the often detrimental ER visits of hospitalization and save CMS some taxpayer money.

You may wonder why a patient would require sub-acute rather than the more intense acute rehab. The discharge planner makes this determination according to how vigorous a program and how many hours of rehab a day the patient can withstand. The planner must do so in accordance with Medicare guidelines. An occasional older patient with a hip fracture or stroke who has a lot of stamina and is highly motivated might be a candidate for the many more hours that acute rehab requires per day.

It also depends how many beds are available. If the acute rehab facility has many open beds, it may take a chance on a borderline patient being eligible for acute care. These facilities tend to be the marquee names in the rehab world (for example, in the Northeast, Kessler, Rusk, etc.) and if one is admitted but cannot keep up with the hours needed, the acute facility can transfer the resident to a locale that specializes in sub-acute care.

There tends to be a lot of competition for Medicare sub-acute patients these days. Facilities often have empty beds and would prefer to fill them with sub-acute residents. The reason for this is mostly financial as we discussed above, though of course the staff enjoys the challenge of getting someone home in better shape than when they came in. Medicare pays the home two to three times the payment they would normally garner for a regular non-rehab resident.

The flip side to this is that the facility needs to know that the resident will cooperate with the program and that he or she has a place to which to be discharged. Alternatively, when the rehab phase is finished, some residents or their families elect to remain long-term and the sub-acute acts as a "feeder" to the long-term care side.

The home will often, but not always, have a nurse or social worker visit the prospective residents in the hospital to see face-to-face if they are appropriate and that the finances are there to pay for long-term care should that become necessary. The nursing home representative will also request the hospital chart records to be certain that sub-acute is appropriate and that correct care can be provided. If the resident needs precautions for a resistant infection, he or she may need a private room. If the patient has serious psychiatric problems, the nursing home needs to know they can handle these professionally and appropriately. The patient and family can also get a first peek into the nursing home by meeting the representative and getting a feel for the place.

Not All Nursing Homes Are Created Equal

Many but not all nursing homes provide sub-acute care. Some are especially geared for it and have a separate wing and nursing staff with that expertise. Others mix the sub-acute residents in with the alert long-term care residents. If your parent is on the younger side and might find being assigned to a nursing unit with older, frailer people distasteful or frightening, then you should opt for a home that has a separate sub-acute unit. As they say, "a picture is worth a thousand words" and I will discuss the visit you should make to see the place for yourself. That should put all these other considerations into perspective.

You will want to be sure that the home is actually licensed by Medicare for sub-acute care and that its reputation is good. Whether the facility is also accredited by JCAHO (Joint Commission on Accreditation of Healthcare Organizations) is, to me, less important. Accreditation may be an additional feather in its cap but should not determine whether or not you use a facility. The JCAHO issue is complicated. The facilities themselves pay for the evaluation and accreditation. The federal powers that be have begun, along with several advocacy groups, to question its utility even in acute care hospitals. Our facility was JCAHO accredited and received a very high score, but we could not justify the financial cost and staff time to repeat the process every few years. The state department of health performs mandatory annual surveys anyway, which are in many cases just as rigorous and get down to nitty-gritty issues.

You will want to know that the home has room for your parent if she needs to stay longer or permanently once the sub-acute care is over. Just as a reminder, Medicare or a Medicare Advantage plan pays for the sub-acute stay. When those twenty to one hundred days expire, who will foot the room-and-board charges, which are substantial? Most, *but not all*, homes accept Medicaid (the government insurance program for the indigent that also pays for daily facility fees) as well as private pay, which means paying out of pocket. If you happen to select a home that is clearly high-end with chandeliers and wall-to-wall carpet and which exudes old-world charm, you may need to pay for all that charm when the rehab stay ends. Again, the home will be delighted to receive lucrative Medicare short-term rehab dollars but flat-out refuse (legally) the miserly Medicaid rate for long-term care. But we have witnessed recently that most homes can no longer refuse Medicaid dollars and survive. A poorly paid bed is better than an empty bed. However, if this is not the case, you may need to transfer your family member to a more reasonably priced place or one that accepts Medicaid once sub-acute care coverage runs out. There are, of course, downsides to such transfers.

The more transfers from one place to another that your family member must endure, the greater the chance for confusion, disorientation, and outright error. The staff at a facility also invests time, energy, and emotion in caring for someone and works hard to hone a plan of care. If you are happy with the care and your parent needs to convert to long-term care, try to stay at the same facility; pick one from the start that will be accommodating. On the other hand, if the sub-acute facility has left you with a bad taste and the staff seems cold and uninterested, consider looking elsewhere. More often than not, these care issues can be worked out. Later in this book I will point out ways to work within the system to improve the care for your family member.

Making Choices

How does one actually choose a place? Word of mouth is extremely important, but please consider the source. While some friends or relatives can be fonts of information and have never steered you wrong, others may mean well but blame a home unfairly. You know and I know that our favorite cousin Marcia may be great company at a family wedding, but has never been satisfied with any restaurant, bakery, or shoe store in the continental United States. Why on earth would she say something nice about a nursing home? Be critical in your questions. Just because someone's second cousin fell at a home within days of being admitted does not mean the home is of poor quality. It could be the home has a progressive attitude toward restraints and allows more freedom and independence. This "empowering" milieu will pay off in the long run in spades and your family member will be happier for it.

Often, one can wangle an off-the-record opinion from the discharge planner. The planner *may* have an ulterior motive in moving you along in your decision and work you like a used car dealer. On the other hand, she may have a sense of professionalism and is in a great position to know the good from the bad and advise you accordingly. You can often use the "if it were your parent, what would you do" line. It works a surprising amount of the time. Look for any flinch or sign of doubt or wavering *and* do your own homework as detailed below.

The quality of a home for the most part remains stable for six-month periods. Your physician could be a good source if you are confident in his or her opinion. Many physicians do not themselves provide care at nursing home rehab centers and can give you an honest opinion of what they've heard from families and other physicians. Some do provide care and will want to steer you to a home at which they have privileges so they can take care of your family member. This may work out well since as the attending physician at the home, the doctor will know the patient and there will be a continuity of care. If you like the care that doctor has provided, then stay with him or her as long as the home has a good reputation. If you were *not* satisfied with the doctor, use this as an opportunity to switch doctors.

Whether for short-term or long-term care, convenience is a major consideration when picking a home. Some prospective residents may have a spouse who is also frail. Driving long distances to visit represents a significant challenge. The ability of a loved one to be on-site and to visit often contributes positively to the care the resident receives. This can be overdone to the point where the family member interferes with the care. It can also be detrimental to the non-institutionalized spouse who may neglect her own well-being to be at the bedside worrying if every medication is given exactly at the correct minute. There exists a fine line between playing a constructive and loving role and becoming trapped in a Joan of Arc syndrome: Martyring oneself to a cause usually helps no one. On balance, it is better to be close enough to visit and to feel that the home welcomes you as a visitor and a partner in care.

Finding and Defining Quality

Convenient visits need to be balanced against finding a good home. If the home nearest you does not measure up, think strongly about another place. Besides word of mouth and a highly recommended visit to see a home for yourself, there is a website called Nursing Home Compare on the Medicare website (www.medicare.gov/ NHCompare), which may help guide you. This is the basis of the so-called "report card" for nursing homes (otherwise known as the Nursing Home Quality Initiative) that began appearing in 2004 as advertisements that Medicare placed in newspapers throughout the country.

Advocacy groups have pressured CMS for years to make the nursing home industry more transparent. One solution was to use hot-button issues that plague long-term care in order to compare different homes. One can read *Consumer Reports* to compare cars or go online to choose the best washing machine, so why not compare nursing homes? After all, they can hold your parent's recovery and life in the balance. Let's take bedsores (pressure ulcers) as an example. Wouldn't you like to know if a certain home has more residents with pressure ulcers than 95% of the other homes in your state? Would it matter to you that a certain home has more residents physically restrained and left in bed than 98% of the other homes in your area? Of course it would—and it should.

Similar report cards exist on the acute care side with, for example, open-heart surgery survival rates. Again, wouldn't you choose a hospital and surgeon whose success rate is 99.99% as opposed to a mere 95% at a second facility? Unfortunately, it's not so simple. The success rate of open-heart surgery may be high at a certain hospital not because their surgeon has the hands of Michelangelo, but because the hospital takes only healthy, "slam-dunk" patients. If you happen to have diabetes and prior heart surgery and are over eighty, they will promptly send you packing. The hospital down the street might take a chance on you even though its statistics might suffer for it. From your point of view, the success rates are meaningless because the first hospital with the gleaming stats would not even give you the time of day. The second hospital, which appeared less desirable, would at least give you a fighting chance. So it is with nursing homes. As a not-for-profit with a mission statement that obligates us to care for those in need regardless of ability to pay, my home routinely accepts residents with complex problems that other homes refuse to consider.

Another problem with quality measures is one of data collection and sample bias. The federal government CMS office bases these measures on self-submitted data from the homes to the government. A report card that just sounds too good to be true may originate from a nursing home with systemic problems submitting its data. Without even being deliberately dishonest, a home can more liberally interpret the CMS quality definitions and make their numbers look better than they really are. For example, it might code a wound on the heel as due to circulation problems when it is really due to pressure, and thus trigger a more positive grade for itself.

I recently heard about a home in our state that had a very low use of restraints and trumpeted that fact widely along with other aspects of its report card. However, on close inspection you'll notice a loophole, which that home seems to have capitalized on. According to the Minimum Data Set that characterizes each individual, for a nursing home resident to be restrained, the restraint must be in place for the prior seven days. This home releases restraints on Sundays for a certain amount of time and then codes these residents as not being restrained. Why Sundays? Sundays in most homes are the busiest day for family members to visit. Friends and families either take the residents out or are by their side so that restraints become unnecessary. There are also group activities, such as music performances, with enough staff in attendance that restraints become superfluous. One could argue that this is good practice on the part of the home since at least it releases the restraints some part of the week. I would believe this if the practice led to restraint reduction on weekdays, too. I have yet to see that this is the case. I think rather that it is an example of how some homes have crafted ways to circumvent the spirit of the Minimum Data Set reports.

The bias issue is important, as we discussed above. A home that has older residents or residents who are admitted from poorer-quality hospitals would likely have higher rates of all negative outcomes. We should praise, not bury, the homes that admit these "tougher" and more challenging residents. Bias can make it hard to assign cause and effect. The reason that nursing homes do not do well on report cards may have nothing to do with poor care. That said, the homes that "fail" their report cards (i.e., are repeatedly worse in their percentile rankings than 90% or more of other homes) likely do have serious problems. I would ask the director of admissions to explain a bad mark and see what he or she tells you. The explanation may be interesting and represent honest grappling with the issue. If the director has a blank look, is not aware of the problem, or cannot even refer you to someone else within the facility, let it be a red flag to you as you wage your battle to find the right home.

The jury may still be out as to whether the tens of websites, thousands of state surveys, and millions of MDS forms have substantively improved long-term care *or* have reduced each home to cookie-cutter similitude. I for one think that in most corners and in most states, long-term care *is* improving and that good homes are rewarded for thinking creatively.

Say Good-bye, Say Hello (Again)

Let's return to the acute care hospital and knowing when to say good-bye. In the race to get you out, the discharge planner may tell you that you have to go to home "x" because "that's the only one with a bed available and you don't have a choice." Do not be cowed by such a statement. If you gently but firmly relate that you need to explore a few places, and in good faith do so over the next few days, most hospitals will agree. The hospital will not want to be in the ugly PR position of moving your family member forcibly. Believe it or not, you may be in the driver's seat.

There may be only one or two nursing homes that are suitable due to geographic issues. You may want your family member admitted to a home with a certain religious or ethnic makeup. There are not-for-profit homes sponsored by Lutherans, Ukrainians, Baptists, Catholics, Chinese, and Jews. In general, not-for-profits tend to be more responsive because one can always appeal to a community board that helps oversee the home (and helps fund the deficits they usually incur).

As to quality of a not-for-profit versus a for-profit home, that is a more difficult call. I have worked at both and tend to think it's a case-by-case proposition. On average, I give an edge to the not-for-profit homes partly because they reinvest any surplus back into the care of the home and not into the shareholders' pockets. There is also a clearer chain of command; one doesn't get the runaround of needing to "check with corporate." In a not-for-profit, where the buck stops is clear.

Some of the for-profits now belong to gargantuan chains and I think their quality and creativity suffer for it. There also tends to be greater turnover in staff, administrators included. I used to admit patients to a facility that was part of a medium-sized for-profit chain. The corporate heads frequently shifted or promoted directors within the system to other homes. The director of nursing seemed to change at least twice a year. Good directors and administrators are hands-on managers and should know their residents and families well. Quick turnover makes this impossible. Nurses and nursing assistants should know their residents better than anyone. High turnover and use of "agency" nurses and aides make this doubly hard. When a nursing home cannot hire enough of its own employee nurses, it may turn to an agency that will send a "nurse du jour" to work an open shift. You should ask if the home uses agency nurses and, if so, how often. Again, the answer should be clear and a high rate of usage is a warning sign.

The vast majority of homes in the country are for-profit so you may not have the luxury of considering a not-for-profit home. The bottom line is that the selection of a home is the resident's and family's choice. You must carefully weigh the decision. At the same time, be fair to the hospital discharge planner or social worker. If you say you need a day or two to make a decision or to visit a home, don't take much more than that. Stalling will not help you and can be harmful to your family member who needs to get on with therapy and the next stage of recovery.

Long-Term Care

If you recall, in the beginning of this chapter I said there were at least two scenarios for your loved one to enter a nursing home. I have focused mainly on scenario number one—the entry from the hospital after medical crisis requires a stay for rehab or close medical care. What if your parent is just not able to live on her own anymore? Perhaps she needs supervision taking her medications or requires help showering and dressing.

The generally accepted guidelines (and in most states requirements if one has Medicaid and the state will be paying for nursing home care) are that an individual is dependent in two or three of the six activities of daily living (referred to as ADLs: the ability to feed, bathe, dress, transfer, toilet oneself, and to remain continent). *Or*, that one can physically perform the activities but due to neurological problems such as dementia can only perform them with supervision. These are the basics but each state has a certifying form that is a bit different and the primary care physician usually completes it.

Remember that there *are* alternatives to nursing homes. One person may require only five minutes of help in dressing to get her shoes on and tied while another may require a good thirty minutes to be fully dressed from top to bottom. Likewise, one person might need her medications lined up in a row with a glass of water but can complete the task herself while another may require each medication to be crushed, mixed with applesauce, and then needs encouragement to swallow.

ASSISTED LIVING

Assisted living facilities (ALFs) can provide help and an alternative to those who are more independent. Usually one pays for the extra help over and above the monthly cost of renting a room. As things change and care needs increase, one can purchase more help. Many assisted living facilities even have separate dementia units, which cater to those with Alzheimer's. Some have medical charts on premises and may or may not have a nurse in twenty-four hour attendance. They all are required to have registered nurse presence for some period of the day. Some provide assistants who can help remind the residents when they need to take their medications but at an extra cost for the help and for the special preparation of the medications.

The ability of each facility to provide care varies greatly. ALFs tend to be more "homey" places with finer and more individualized cuisine, but quality can vary significantly. Most states require a license but regulations vary among states and over time. Most of those who live in ALFs pay privately and it is usually cheaper than nursing home care. The difference is that if one qualifies for Medicaid (a big *if*), the nursing home might cost very little since Medicaid covers nursing home care. Some states have ALF waivers. These fund a limited number of Medicaid recipients to live in ALFs, but such funding and rooms are hard to come by. The AARP has a nice checklist of questions to ask if you visit an ALF. Visit www.aarp.org/families/health/, click on Long-Term Care, and then look for the Checklist: Evaluating Assisted-Living Facilities.

OTHER CHOICES

There are other even more independent settings like foster homes and group homes for seniors that are springing up all over the country. There is government-subsidized senior housing (known as Section 202 housing and overseen by HUD). Vermont has an interesting program that will *pay* family members to care for their own Medicaid-receiving elderly relatives…always taboo before, but Vermont sees it as a win-win. It saves money on the cost of a nursing home and the individual is happier remaining at home.

How do you know what level of care is necessary? You need to assess what your loved one can do and what she needs help in doing. You may live with her presently and know that information well. If you don't, it behooves you to consult a professional. Your family doctor may have experience in the different levels of care and steer you in the right direction. A social worker with expertise in the field or a geriatric care manager will know the ups and downs of the different options available. If the care needs are not great, he or she might be able to tell you how to avail your-selves of services that will keep your loved one at home. There are many ways to search for a geriatric care manager near you by using either the phone book or the Internet. One website to visit is www.caremanager.org, but there are several.

You may be able to get a quick and cheap assessment done by a physical or occupational therapist who has been seeing your parent for some other reason such as a shoulder or knee problem. The therapist may have experience in long-term care and recommend the proper setting. The important message is that if you have any doubts, please do everyone a favor and be sure they really *need* a nursing home. If you do visit an alternative facility, many of the same principles from this book can be applied. My two caveats are:

1) If your loved one is very old and very frail, and it is a border-line call that they can make it at an assisted living facility, think ahead of how distressing and time-consuming *another* move will be if she flunks out of assisted living. Any single

move can be traumatic, but two moves close together is a *lot* to handle.

2) Assisted living facilities have been largely overbuilt and therefore have empty beds. They have a financial incentive to fill their beds. A particular facility may be reluctant to recommend transfer to a nursing home even when your parent needs much more help than it can safely provide. Remember, many assisted living facilities do *not* have any nurses during the evenings and nights.

Ultimately, you will make the choice so look around and get good advice up front.

The Internet has a plethora of information on long-term care. A nice resource is the American Association of Homes and Services for the Aging. This group and its state affiliates represent close to 6,000 not-for-profit homes. The website is www.aahsa.org. Click on Consumer Information for useful information on nursing homes and ALFs in your area. If your loved one is a veteran, see the Veterans Administration website www.va.gov and click on FAQs, and then search for nursing homes. Medicare also has information on choosing a nursing home and what Medicare covers. Try www.medicare.gov. Click on Long-Term Care on the left.

Summary of Chapter 1

- Does your family member need long-term care coming from home, or sub-acute care (Medicare Part A, skilled care) coming from a hospital?

- If coming from home, is a nursing home necessary or would an alternative such as assisted living or increased home services be suitable? Can the physician, geriatric care manager, or social worker help you with the decision?

- If coming from the hospital, is sub-acute rehab care appropriate or might your family member qualify for more strenuous acute rehab? Don't be cowed by an aggressive discharge planning staff. Does the physician approve the discharge? Has status of tubes, oxygen, medications, etc., been determined?

- Take extra time to visit (within reason) and try to pick the right place the first time. Does the home accept Medicaid (even if only for future reference)? Is a bed available now?

- If your family member is younger or would feel uncomfortable in a nursing home, is there a separate sub-acute unit that might cater better to her needs?

- Assess the importance to you of geographic proximity to your home.

- Consider advice on your choice from physicians, social workers, hospital personnel, and friends. Consult www.medicare.gov/NHCompare for free (or other sites requiring a fee). Ask for a tour.

- Consider how important a religious or ethnically based home is to your loved one.

2

The Tour: Can We Talk?

Let's say you still don't have an absolute feel for what home is right and there is no geographic imperative. Strongly consider making a field trip to visit one or a few homes. If you have siblings or other family members who wish to be involved, as many as possible should visit at the same time. One of you may notice something that another misses. If things also eventually go wrong, you don't want to be blamed or start blaming each other. A home should be happy to give you a tour; if it is not, I would avoid that home. Call the director of admissions and schedule a visit.

The home will ask you to fill out an application. This will include important health information and a history of prior medical care; it should also pose questions that allow you to describe your parent as a person. Is she outgoing or does she prefer privacy? Can she participate in discussion groups? What are her hobbies? Does she harbor strong likes and dislikes for certain kinds of food, music, people? You will likely be asked for some financial information. While it may seem intrusive and you might be reluctant to divulge, this will help the home determine how your loved one will pay for her stay. Does she have Medicaid already or will she soon qualify for it after "spending down" her own money? Does she have private long-term care insurance? Look upon this exercise not as intrusive but as educational. Ask the staff how they can assist you in planning for the future and accessing funds or how to apply for Medicaid if that is in the cards.

If your parent is alert and can cooperate, by all means include him or her in completing the application and making the visit. There are several things you will want to know from the director when you meet with him or her.

Asking Questions

- *Is there a bed available right away or is there a waiting list?* While waiting lists can indicate a popular and sought-after home, they are largely a thing of the past. There are too many alternatives and there is too much competition for there to be a seller's market. However, while a home may not be full, it may have only a certain number of beds slated for sub-acute care and one may not be immediately available. The bed should also be on a nursing unit or wing that is appropriate. Your parent's level of alertness and ability should match that of most residents on that nursing unit. The better homes are large enough so that comparable residents live on the same unit. An alert seventy-year-old who needs reconditioning in order to return home should not share a room with an agitated ninety-nine-year-old who is dying of pneumonia. There may also be infectious disease issues. If your parent picked up a particular infection that requires *precautions* (formerly known as *isolation*), she will probably need a private room, which might not be immediately available.

A good nursing home may have only one or two beds available and the placement of your parent may not be ideal. What to do? One could ask the admissions director of the home to confer with the discharge planner at the hospital and beg for a few more days until a more appropriate bed opens up. This may not work. More likely you will need to choose the lesser of two evils. If the home is really terrific and you have ample reason to want your family member there, I would agree to the bed, transfer your family member to the home, and tough it out for a few days. A better bed should open up soon. If the home's admission director cannot be pinned down to a move within the facility in four or five days, then I would regrettably look elsewhere. If elsewhere turns out to be "the land that time forgot," you can always try to have your family member transferred over to your first choice when an appropriate bed opens up.

- *What is the therapy schedule and who are the therapists?* Many homes contract with a local or national therapy group to provide services. Some employ therapists of their own. It will be hard for you to judge which one is better, but if a local hospital or acute rehab center with a good reputation provides the therapists, it's a good bet that they will be competent and well trained. The other advantage is that they will provide substitutes if the usual therapist is away. There is more turnover with these larger groups but the sub-acute stays are short enough that it should not be a concern. At our home, the short-term rehab therapists have each been with us for many years and are warm, talented, and conscientious; they know our population well. For our other therapies, known in the business as "Part B" (as in Medicare Part B, which pays for some outpatient therapy), we contract with a national group.

The therapists are also terrific, but the turnover is a bit too high for my tastes. On the other hand, when a therapist is out sick or on vacation, we never have to cancel a therapy session.

Therapy on weekends used to be a luxury but it *should* be available at least one weekend day. The better homes provide this (which, by the way, beats most acute care hospitals). The main point is to be sure you visit the therapy room during your visit; find out in advance when you are likely to see the most action there and plan your visit accordingly. The therapists should be energetic, lively, and proud of their work. You might want to engage one of them in conversation and tell them a bit about your family member. While the therapists may be on the busy side, this is a quick way to get a feel for the department.

- *What are the opportunities for family meetings to discuss progress?* The staff should schedule family meetings within the first few weeks and certainly at least a week before anticipated discharge. If the social worker balks at this question or is unsure how to answer, it may signify a staff that is none too helpful. There will also be times when *you* want to call a meeting as the need arises. One can sometimes handle issues by speaking to an individual staff person. For example, if you want to see your mom back on an antidepressant that for some reason was stopped in the hospital, you should call the attending physician. If the attending does not respond to your call, then notify the medical director or administrator of the home. That should do the trick. On the other hand, if you are unclear whether your family member can go home or should go to assisted living, a family meeting would be the best venue to get all the team members' input. Consensus from the team is important on decisions as far-reaching as this.

- *What are the opportunities to stay after the rehab period if discharge home is not feasible?* The fewer moves your parent makes, the better. Will he or she remain on the same unit or move elsewhere once therapy is complete? If the answer to the second part is yes, then by all means be sure that other unit is included in your tour. Many facilities now have a separate area for sub-acute rehab. They tend to be the newer and nicer parts in a home. The homes may house long-term residents elsewhere and, in the words of the *Michelin Guide*, it is "worth a detour" to see it for yourself.

- *How are the units divided and are there any special units for dementia?* Good homes group their residents according to mental and physical function. They care about the emotional comfort of the residents and see them as individuals who need to interact and develop relationships with other individuals. Some homes may be too small to accomplish this. That is not a flat-out negative, but the other aspects of care would have to be darn good to make up for it. A home that has a specially accredited Alzheimer's or dementia unit usually is a progressive, forward-looking place. These units demand a higher level of training and staffing and even though you may not be interested in it now, it's nice to know it's there.

- *How does one choose a doctor?* You should be wary of a home that does not have a transparent procedure for choosing a physician. This doesn't mean you will always be able to choose the doctor you think you want, but the way in which the home organizes the medical staff tells a lot about it. The discussion should be open and you should feel free to at least get the name and phone number of the physician who may be assigned. You should be able to choose from a few different doctors but with the following caveat: Many of the best homes have adopted a "closed" staff model, which means there are only a few physicians who work there. They tend to be specialists in geriatrics and may even have fellowship training and/or board qualifications in that field. This is a good sign and the fact that your parent is assigned to one of these doctors should improve their care. Having fewer doctors implies that each doctor cares for many of the residents in the home and consequently is there almost daily.

Our home has four doctors for about three hundred residents and each is trained and certified in geriatrics. Because of the large responsibility this entails, each doctor makes rounds four or five days a week and has chosen to make long-term care a central part of his or her practice. If one of the physicians is not available on a certain day, there is always another one at the home who can "cover." I have also worked at homes with large "open" medical staffs. An open medical staff model means that any physician who wishes may admit his patient to that home and care for her during the stay. The home chooses this model because it wants to cast a wide net for referrals. All too often, however, the doctors in the open model have only a handful of patients and visit once or twice a month. The rest are handled by phone or with an order to evaluate a problem in the local emergency room.

While your family doctor who has cared for your parent for years may be happy to follow him or her into the nursing home, she may not have the time, interest, or training to do so properly. Many veteran docs think that "anyone" can care for a nursing home patient. I'm afraid this is less true with each passing year. Long-term care is practically a specialty unto itself. If a closed staff model does not exist, you should ask for a doctor who comes in to make rounds often, at least several times a week. Better yet, ask at the hospital for recommendations as to which doctors at a certain home enjoy good reputations. If a certain doctor is outstanding and your parent has complex medical issues, it may even be worth choosing a home because that doctor attends there.

You should feel confident that the doctor you choose is skilled and interested in nursing home residents. He or she may not get back to you immediately when you call with a question. Barring extenuating circumstances, however, you should hear back within a day or two. If that doesn't happen or you simply feel uncomfortable with the doctor, you have the right to ask for a change. While visiting your parent, you may even have noticed a physician who is frequently present and seems to have a nice manner. The nurses or nursing assistants may take you into their confidence and tell you the doctor's name or recommend someone else.

Each home has a medical director who is usually present more than the other doctors. If that person is well thought of, he or she might be a good bet. Caveat emptor: Occasional medical directors are not particularly attuned to nursing home care and may have received the appointment as a favor or even because they are the administrator's private physician (or golf partner). This will likely change as CMS cracks down on the position and ensures responsibility and accountability. Check to see if the director is a CMD (certified medical director) by the AMDA (American Medical Directors Association). This is a sign of significant training and commitment and should allay most fears. Again the *key* factor is the willingness of the director of admissions to divulge as much information as will be helpful to you. Anything short of that augurs poorly for the home.

Summary of Chapter 2

- Schedule a tour with siblings present (if possible). If the spouse of the patient or the patient is available, all the better (if appropriate).

- How does the home categorize residents on the nursing units or wings (i.e., by functional and/or cognitive abilities)? Is a bed available on a unit that suits your family member?

- If a bed is not available on the proper unit, how long until one becomes available and what are the pros and cons of a temporary placement on another unit?

- Is the sub-acute unit separate and what amenities are included (phone, TV, etc.)? Is it clean and does staff make eye contact and chat easily?

- Visit the therapy room. Is the staff energetic and interactive? Do the therapists call residents by name? Is there at least one day of weekend therapy?

- Visit the unit to which your family member would be transferred if he/she cannot return home. Is there a noticeable divergence between this unit and the sub-acute? Is there a separate Alzheimer's or dementia unit with specially trained staff (even if you don't need it presently)?

- Is the medical staff small or large? Can you pick your own doctor? Are any of the doctors certified medical directors (CMDs) or members of AMDA? Do any of them have added qualifications (boards) in geriatrics?

3

The Tour and Beyond:
Now Let's Walk

You have a list of homes or perhaps one home that fits the bill. The geographic location is acceptable. You have met with the director of admissions and asked many of the questions discussed in chapter 2. Now tour the facility with the director or the director's designee. If you are with other family members, you might place different priorities on aspects of care, but try to present a united front. The nursing home will also get a sense that you are a family that wants to remain involved and cater to you a bit differently. If you simply make decisions better on your own or are an only child, then proceed accordingly. Most important is your gut reaction while walking through the home.

What to Look For

Almost all homes have a lobby and a receptionist that provide you with an immediate impression of the facility. Is the lobby clean, bright, and well maintained? The administration knows that many people judge a book by its cover and if it doesn't keep the lobby at least attractive and clean, then one would have to wonder about the rest of the home. Notice I did not say the lobby should knock your socks off. I've seen several new homes with lobbies that are right out of *Architectural Digest*, but when you scratch the surface, the care is marginal. These tend to be the larger chains that have cookie-cutter designs for each facility. The owners know that a glittering chandelier will grab your attention and divert your eye from the underside if there is one.

The receptionist should be friendly and helpful. The receptionist is the first person anyone meets and for better or for worse puts a stamp on the home. His or her phone manners are also key in presenting the facility in a positive light. Everyone is entitled to a bad day, but a persistently crabby or rude receptionist speaks volumes about the home. You will have plenty of contact with the receptionist, who will transfer your calls and greet you each time you visit. Do not be surprised if the receptionist is sorting papers or filing envelopes while doing her reception work. Most homes run on a tight budget so a receptionist who is responsible for other tasks is acceptable. He or she should be cheerful when helping you, making sure you are directed the correct way in the home. If something seems amiss, ask if the person at the desk is the regular receptionist and judge accordingly.

Most homes these days, like most businesses, tout customer satisfaction as a mantra for success. They should be training the staff to answer phones politely and "own" problems until they are solved. If the receptionist has not adopted a helpful demeanor, then you may have to worry about the aides and nurses, too. The receptionist is, in a sense, the touchstone of the entire staff; a good one goes a long way.

As you walk through the halls, think of T. S. Eliot's line from the poem "The Love Song of J. Alfred Prufrock": "To prepare a face to meet the faces that you meet." Does the staff smile and make eye contact easily? While not everyone loves their work and certainly many of us have bad days, the staff should display some sense of camaraderie and élan. Also crucial is observing how staff members interact with residents. Are they respectful? Do they address them directly, perhaps even leaning over to speak close to their ear or right in front of them if they have trouble hearing or seeing? It is not as important whether they address the resident as "Mr." or "Mrs." or by first name, but a sense of caring should permeate the home.

When I refer to staff members here, I mean not only the nurses or nursing assistants, though they are in many ways the key staff. The housekeepers and maintenance workers, too, should have a kind and respectful demeanor to the residents. If you've spent much time in a nursing home, you know that the housekeepers and maintenance crew are almost denizens of the home as they pass in and out of rooms, halls, and dining areas every day. They become like family to the residents. In a good home, this is encouraged and even formalized. One of our older maintenance staff members happens to be a musician in his spare time. It is not uncommon to find him accompanying the resident's choir when our regular pianist is out. At our home, and many homes that are adopting a new philosophy known as "culture change" (see box on p. 37), we train these staff members to participate regularly with residents in activities such as bingo, music, and exercise.

You will also want to observe that the top brass knows the residents by name and is solicitous of them. Administrators who are not may be equally diffident when problems arise later on. I love an administrator who relates seemingly trivial but very human

Culture Change

There is a phenomenon known as "culture change," which, if not quite sweeping long-term care, is taking hold in some pockets. Most good homes are at least adopting facets of its philosophy. Put simply, the culture change movement insists that nursing homes should accent the "home" and de-emphasize the "nursing." In culture change the home environment is paramount. That could mean letting pets roam the hallways or allowing a resident to cook his own corn dog at three in the morning if he has a craving—cholesterol levels be damned! Groups such as the Eden Alternative led by Dr. William Thomas (www.edenalt.org) and the Pioneer Network (www.pioneernetwork.net) exemplify this approach. It is worth visiting these websites to get a taste of culture change and to glimpse the future of long-term care.

details about residents and families. If the tour leader stops to tell you a story about a certain resident who you run into, or shows some pride in someone who learned to walk again after therapy, this is a sign of a humane and caring home and leader. My chaplain in medical school taught me that the secret to providing good care for a patient is to care *about* the patient and that holds true in long-term care. Look for it on your tour. I recently overheard our executive director arranging for a resident to get a ride to her favorite hairdresser while her son was away. In fact, I wouldn't have been surprised if he ended up driving her himself. As they say in baseball, that won't show up in the box score, but it certainly wins games.

Be sure to see the nursing unit that is proposed for your family member. Many homes, or at least the larger ones, group the residents according to both physical and mental function. This benefits the resident. It is rare for a "with it" and alert resident to prefer to be on a unit where the majority of the residents are forgetful and confused. I do have an occasional resident who subscribes to the "big fish in a small pond" theory of life and who is relieved by *not* having to interact with other alert residents. By and large, though, you will want your family member to be with like-minded people who she can befriend and with whom she can feel comfortable.

On the other hand, you *will* want your confused family member with dementia to be with others that suffer from the same problem. The staff on these units is usually more tolerant and accepting of the resident; the expectations are not as high. While in a school-age child you may not *want* to lower expectations, in a frail person with dementia the demands of a "higher"-functioning unit will be too much. It places stress on the person and results in anxiety and worsening behavior. I have also seen alert residents look down on (in the best case) and actually torment (in the worst case) disoriented and forgetful residents. Some of this is born of fear and not of maliciousness, but the result is the same.

When you examine the unit, be sure to meet the head nurse and some of his or her staff. Does the head nurse interact well and make eye contact with you? She is a key player and if you take an instant shine to her, it may signify good things to come. The head nurse on a unit is the director and should be able to expect and achieve good work habits from all her staff. As you will realize, the nursing assistants are the main actors with regard to hands-on physical care but also are the ones who engage the residents the most. The ideal head nurse understands the plight of having to do backbreaking work for little pay, yet must be firm enough to ensure that the care is delivered—over and over again. She must be a problem solver and innovator who is flexible enough to work with you when you have new ideas, but who can also create them herself. See more about key personnel in chapter 5.

If there are any vacant rooms, ask to see them. When you pick a hotel room for a vacation, you would most likely look at pictures online. Take the same interest here. While it would be great to have your choice regarding a single or a double, there may be homes with few options and you won't have your pick. It is not a foregone conclusion that a single is preferable. Some residents need and crave privacy while others are social and like the idea of a room-mate. I used to work in a VA hospital that still had large rooms of between four to eight people. Contrary to what you might expect, many of the veterans liked the bigger rooms because there was more activity and more people with whom to interact. They often looked out for each other and if there were good pairings, the salu-tary effect was priceless. The disadvantage in sharing a room is that today's nursing homes frequently turn over (euphemism for death or being discharged to a hospital). Today's "good neighbor Sam" could turn into tomorrow's resident from hell. Private rooms usually cost more and some homes save them for infection con-trol reasons. Some homes don't have any private rooms and some few have only private rooms. Above all, the room should be clean with some ventilation. Ask to see the heating and air-conditioning units to be sure they are working. Many homes have individual units, which is great because many elderly residents prefer a range between eighty to ninety degrees! If there are not individual units, don't sweat it because other things can be more important.

The Nitty-Gritty: Time to Apply

If you are serious about the home, you will most likely be asked to fill out an application and other paperwork. Some of this will be insurance information and financial clarification of what is covered or not by Medicare and/or Medicaid. Be sure to bring all information you might have in regard to secondary insurance plans. These are often known as Medigap policies and include plans from major insurance companies as well as AARP. If the stay is purely for long-term care, you will have to discuss finances in more detail.

With the advent of the Medicare Part D prescription plan, it behooves you to bring your membership card to show to what PDP (prescription drug plan) your family member belongs. As long as you are on sub-acute, Medicare Part A pays for your drugs. As soon as you are off sub-acute and you either return to your community or remain for long-term care, you will be back on Medicare Part D. If you stay at the home, find out from the home or the pharmacy supplier which PDPs are oriented to long-term care and participate with that pharmacy. The home should have a list of these plans and you can pick freely from them. Unfortunately, the switch may not happen until the first of the next month. Medicare is still working out some of the Part D kinks but it is saving people money. However, expect to have greater difficulty obtaining brand-name medications—as opposed to generics—under Part D.

If your family member has significant assets, you will likely need to declare them in a worksheet. The home justifiably needs to know that they can count on payment for services provided. The time to have consulted an eldercare lawyer to transfer assets to others (usually the adult children) is long past and most states are making these rules even more stringent. The "look-back" period in many states is three years, which means that money transferred within three years to a relative or friend is fair game. It still counts toward assets you must spend down. It will take you that much longer to qualify for room and board under Medicaid.

The Johnson administration did not create Medicaid to pay for nursing home care. It has over the decades become the payer of "last resort" for long-term care. When one has spent down and no longer has assets to pay for care, then one can apply to Medicaid. The kicker is that even without assets, monthly income from a pension, annuity, and/or social security can be great enough to preclude Medicaid benefits. The house your family member may own is always a question mark but most states will allow the remaining spouse to keep the house without it counting as an asset. This does vary from state to state and as budgets tighten, one can expect changes. Again, recall that this is for long-term care and not the short-stay sub-acute rehab that Medicare covers regardless of assets.

Despite the difficulty in transferring assets at this point, it may still be worth a few hours to consult a qualified eldercare lawyer to be sure that everything that could still be put in order *is* put in order for the application. As long as you are at it, talk about the other parent for whom you may need advice down the road. You will not achieve anything by being secretive about assets; the state will figure it out when you apply for Medicaid. To find a reputable eldercare lawyer try word of mouth, consult the yellow pages, or go to the web. There are thousands of these lawyers now in the country and a search in your area should turn one up quickly.

Elder law attorneys may belong to the National Academy of Elder Law Attorneys. The group's website is www.naela.com. It will assist you in finding a reputable attorney in your area either by experience in the different realms of elder law and/or by certification as a Certified Elder Law Attorney (CELA). There are some fine elder law attorneys without this certification, but certification means that the attorney devotes a significant amount of time to elder law and has passed a six-hour examination. Another excellent source of information is the website Elder Law Answers at www.elderlawanswers.com, which can help you find an elder lawyer *and* is a rich source of information for the layperson.

You may also be asked for medical information from your family member's private physician. This information coupled with the hospital records will help the physician and team who ultimately care for your family member. The home will also determine in each case if it can provide adequate care. For example, very few nursing homes accept residents on a ventilator. Those few that do must have special equipment and a highly trained staff. Some nursing homes carry out a type of dialysis called peritoneal dialysis. The staff performs this at the bedside of the patient several times a day but it obviates the need to travel to a dialysis center three times a week for hemodialysis. Even if a nursing home does not currently perform the procedure, it might be willing to learn as ours did several years ago. Don't be frightened off by your family member being the first person in the facility to undergo a certain procedure or treatment. If the director of nursing and the medical staff are willing to learn, it shows a flexibility and curiosity that bodes well for the place. You should get a quick sense if the director of nursing or his or her staff are rigid "Nurse Ratcheds." The nursing profession spearheads much of the reform that is blossoming in long-term care in this country and it would be a shame to be involved with a home that is not part of the movement.

Timing the Tour/Testing the Waters

You should ask for a morning tour if possible; in most homes, you will see more activity in the early hours than in the afternoon. Observe mealtimes if you can. It is important to note how many of the residents are out of their rooms for meals. Nearly all homes should have residents in the dining area for each meal. There are always a few "refuseniks" who, no matter what, prefer to eat in their own room and technically have the right to do so. There will also be a smattering of residents who are in bed due to illness, infection control issues, or the need to give them a rest from constantly being in a chair.

Having the residents up and out of bed is one of the salient features that distinguishes long-term care from acute care. Acute care hospitals are notorious for letting patients wallow in their beds. The unwitting victims become easy prey for bedsores, dysphagia (poor ability to swallow), and pneumonia. Some places are more tuned in than others and more power to them. But few are as tuned in as even your most retro nursing home.

And try eating while lying in bed even if your head is at about thirty degrees elevation, which is what happens at most hospitals. It is patently dangerous. Every day when I make rounds at the hospital I find patients at a terrible angle with an unopened food tray sadly out of reach and no one in the room to help. When I make rounds with residents (young doctors in training), the first thing we do is to adjust the head of the bed, open the food containers, and feed the patients. At least then we are doing some good. Many hospitals these days do not orient themselves to the commonsense needs of the frail, elderly patient. Some are so busy hiring star chefs to manage their food program and concierges for the front desk that the basics are lost in the shuffle.

At the nursing home there may be a unit with very alert individuals who need no assistance at all. These units do exist at certain homes but have become rare indeed. The assisted living phenomenon has siphoned off the more alert and independent residents, and most of those who reside in a nursing home need supervision if not direct assistance. Be sure there appears to be enough help to ensure adequate intake for the residents. Some residents eat very slowly. I once cared for a particular gentleman who rode a Harley well into his eighties. As he aged into his nineties, he slowed down but maintained his dignity and dressed in a jacket and tie for every meal. I remember that he came into the home with his wife and though we asked him if they would like a double room, he chose separate rooms, winked at me, and whispered, "Enough is enough." He would take a full three hours to consume breakfast and would just be finishing when the lunch trolleys arrived. The Italians say that no one grows old while sitting at a meal and perhaps he took this to heart.

There is nothing wrong with eating that slowly and a good home should make adjustments and be flexible. But a resident who is just staring at a meal, and no one provides help, can be a bad sign indeed. Portions tend to be large and very few frail elders can complete a full meal. Therefore, food left on the plate does not imply poor care. The more eyes and ears and hands on deck for breakfast the better; it is often the most well-received meal of the day. Good homes will recruit all available staff to help feed the residents. This might include nurses, aides, activity therapists, social workers, and even paid "feeders." When I have spare time, and especially during snowstorms when staff is late, I enjoy feeding residents myself. It is a golden opportunity to see how they function and how they interact with others; besides, it just makes me feel good.

Feeding Tubes and End-of-Life Care

If the nursing home you visit contains large numbers of feeding tubes, you should be wary. You might even ask how many feeding tubes are present. You can also find the number on the CMS website (www.cms.hhs.gov/). Our home has an unusually low rate of about 4%. If more than 10% of a home's residents have feeding tubes, it may indicate a troubling philosophy of care.

The feeding tube issue will come up later in a discussion on end-of-life care and nutrition, but some nursing homes will opt for feeding tubes out of convenience or to achieve a financial advantage. However, tubes don't necessarily mean bad care and perhaps they service a population that, due to religious reasons or ethnic tradition, demands these appliances.

You should ask the tour guide about the home's philosophy regarding feeding tubes and end-of-life care. You will want to hear an answer that is consonant with your beliefs. If you are a right-to-lifer and believe in feeding tubes and aggressive care to the bitter end, then look for a similarly minded staff. Contrarily, and representing the majority of residents and families, if you believe in death with dignity and comfort being a priority, then look for a staff that reflects and encourages these values.

There are still some nursing homes and physicians who insist a permanent artificial feeding tube be placed when a resident stops eating. They can pressure you in all kinds of subtle and not-so-subtle ways. It is unclear that these homes and doctors have the right to do this; it could well be worth a legal battle if you have the stomach for it. If not, then pick a home that believes what you believe. Several years ago, a family asked me to transfer a very old but adored and accomplished family member with advanced Alzheimer's from a nursing home to a hospital, essentially to let her die. It was a home with a policy of mandatory feeding tubes and did not believe in less aggressive forms of care such as hospice.

At that time, a home was allowed to do this as long as they sought alternative places for families who objected to their philosophy. I would hope at this point that such places are few in number. It was a very sad and needless end to an otherwise distinguished life.

While you're at it, ask about hospice care, which I will discuss more fully in the last chapter. Very briefly, hospice is an approach to caring for those whose life expectancy for whatever reason is less than six months (whether from cancer, Alzheimer's, emphysema, etc.). It focuses on comfort, pain control, and dignity. CMS has estimated that 10–15% of nursing home residents are appropriate for hospice care. If the home you are visiting does not even have a contract with a hospice agency or only 1 or 2% of the residents are on hospice, it may indicate a philosophy that doesn't accept the hospice comfort-care approach. For most, that would be a major negative. Lack of hospice services implies a backward-thinking staff and administration. Hospice and palliative care alternatives are the way of the future in long-term care and, in my estimation, facilities are foolish not to avail themselves of these services. Some homes avoid hospice for specious financial reasons and to avoid potential litigation. The longer the home can keep someone alive or fed by a tube, the longer they can bill Medicaid or the family for the stay.

Observe and Engage

Get a sense of the food and the ability of the place to deliver hot meals to all the units in a timely way. The dining areas should be centers of activity. Between meals they are often used for activities and family visits. Some homes have auditoriums, solariums, or atriums that fill this role, and the dining rooms are reserved for eating. That is fine, but the point is that for some part of the day, these rooms should bustle with activity. A home without a sense of life might house its residents too much in their rooms. "And what's wrong with that?" you might ask. Residents, of course, have the right to stay in their rooms. Some choose even to eat their meals in their rooms. At a good home, though, such citizens are few and far between. In our home of three hundred residents there are two residents who remain almost wholly in their rooms. There may be another thirty who would rather stay in their rooms but who can be persuaded or encouraged to socialize and participate in activities with other residents. The vast majority is happy to be with others and recognize (or their families recognize) the benefits of being out and about.

Though it can vary widely depending on what level unit one visits, I would also note how the residents respond to you. If the residents on the unit you visit are debilitated and dependent, ask to see a more alert unit. On such a unit, there should be some spirit and passion. The staff should be paying attention to the residents and not watching television. At our home we have a rule that televisions stay off during mealtime. While it is not easy to enforce this, we do it so the staff engages the residents. If the residents appear down or are not chatting with each other, they may not be getting the help and TLC they deserve.

Stop and chat with a few residents. Beware if the tour leader discourages you or moves you along. I will temper this by saying that nursing homes often attract difficult residents, some of whom are there because they have alienated and exhausted their own family members. You may well run into a resident who is confused, delusional, paranoid, or constantly asking for help. You could ask the tour guide for an explanation and listen carefully to the answer. Within the constraints of confidentiality, the guide should try to explain the situation to you. If you remain baffled, don't let it deter you; nursing homes can be difficult places in which to live or to visit. Residents on lower-functioning units can be needy and noisy. I would be more concerned about a higher-functioning unit that has a resident who is babbling, paranoid, or downright disruptive and to whom the staff does not respond.

A good rule of thumb is that if you observe a difficult situation, ask for an explanation. The words the guide chooses and the actions the guide displays will speak volumes about the culture of the home. The representatives of the home should speak as directly and clearly to the residents as they would to you. If in front of a guest they are disrespectful to a resident, one can only imagine what the interactions are when no one is there as a witness.

A story comes to mind of a nursing home near us that was undergoing a state survey. The inspectors noted that a nurse went into a room without knocking. This is a major no-no and for good reason. You would certainly not want people entering your home without knocking or announcing who they are. The room of a nursing home resident is his or her home no matter how small or bare or antiseptic it may look. Unless there is a good reason to enter, it should be inviolable to outsiders. This sacred right to privacy often used to be overlooked in nursing homes. Thanks to the nursing home reform movement and the now enshrined "resident's rights," it no longer is.

The state further investigated this particular home and found that *no one* knocked when entering a room—even during a state survey! One can only imagine what it was like without the survey team present. The team concluded that if there was such disregard for a fundamental right like privacy, there were likely to be even less savory things going on. They decided to make a statement to the home and to the industry by closing the facility to new admissions. This was a home that was barely making it financially; new admissions are the lifeblood of such a place. The state forced them to devise an action plan to remedy the situation. They did so and the improvement spilled over into every facet of the home. The disregard for residents was plowed under and the home did well on the next several surveys. That's an example of the survey system working at its best. Unfortunately, not all surveys are so constructive or end as well, but there are signs of hope.

Let's get back to our tour. Learn as much as you can by the interactions you observe and ask those who accompany you how they view the home. Again try to look beyond the glitz or the gloom. What are the most telling features of the staff and do you feel comfortable enough to entrust your loved one to its care? You may want to come back and sit in the lobby or spend part of your time after the tour reading the paper and soaking up the atmosphere. You'll be able to see a myriad of interactions and get a flavor for the place. Good leadership can achieve the kind of behavior and dedication that one wants to see in a facility that cares for the frailest among us. Honesty on the part of the staff is the best and most welcome policy for a home. It will inform every interaction you have with the nurses, doctors, therapists, and even the business office. There are few perfect homes; you will have to make concessions along the way. But if the *handpicked* representatives of the home are not forthcoming on the tour, you should be on your guard and consider other places.

It is unlikely that you'll be able to taste the food, but at least look at a menu to check for variety and see if alternative choices exist. This will also help inform you as to the flexibility of the home. Older people can be notoriously difficult when it comes to food so take their comments with a large amount of salt!

In the last twenty years, many homes have adopted a system whereby workers on a line in the kitchen place food on a tray. It is then transported via heating trolleys to each unit. A favorite way for state surveyors to bust chops, as it were, is to measure the temperature of food delivered by cart. The home can earn a deficiency if the food is tepid rather than hot.

Homes with "off-tray service" feature a better dining experience. Rather than delivering the food to the table on trays assembled on a production line, the staff serves the meals individually from chafing dishes. Though the food is not necessarily tastier, the ambience is almost always nicer. In an effort to be truly homey, some sport fancy linen and fine silver. They manage to evoke memories of a gilded age. Think of the dinner scenes with Judy Garland in *Meet Me in St. Louis* and you'll understand what I mean. In channeling the past, homes with off-tray service manage to be a step ahead. Because it is so demanding in terms of staff time, setup, and clearing, homes often limit fancier service to the more alert floors. These homes should be commended just for attempting something new. We have instituted it on several of our units and it has not been easy, but the feedback is positive.

Signs of Life

Good homes distinguish themselves from hospitals by pushing residents to get out of bed. I am shocked by how reluctant the staff is, even at some very good hospitals, to get patients out of bed. As a physician, I can write all the orders I want, but unless a nursing staff has the interest or can rally enough help, it never gets done. This is why pressure ulcers (bedsores) are so common in our hospitals. I have admitted immobilized patients who remained without sores for years in our home and yet develop them in a mere three days in the hospital. The hospital is quick to enlist the help of a wound-care nurse once the sore has developed, but is loathe to invest in the basic tenets of prevention that are the currency of most nursing homes.

I recently cared for an alert but frail woman who told me that in the week she was hospitalized, she was not once taken out of bed to sit in a chair. I'd like to think this is the exception, but it is still too common. When I enter a hospital room, I often find my patient trying to feed herself while more horizontal than vertical in bed. Much of the food spills onto the bedclothes as the patient coughs or chokes. She loses her dignity *and* is at risk for pneumonia. Talk about a recipe for disaster. Nursing homes look great by comparison. Until some of these hospitals improve, such misdirected care behooves us to keep a sick older person out of the hospital if possible.

There are some wonderful hospitals with leadership staff that gets it, but many do not. *So,* be sure the residents you see on your tour are out of bed and in common areas. On heavier care units, the residents often return to bed after lunch in order to rest or to nap, which is perfectly acceptable. Morning visits are therefore better, but if you have no choice, remember to ask about anything you might see that seems amiss.

Ask to see a calendar of events and activities and look at it carefully with your family member if he or she is able. Each unit should have a blackboard that lists the day's activities and it should be updated often. There should be at least one or two activities per day, even on units with severely impaired residents. Though severely demented and debilitated residents may not seem to absorb much, the activities are key to maintaining whatever abilities remain. They also help occupy the residents and decrease the number of drugs that would otherwise be used to sedate or chemically restrain them. The activities should not be all bingo all the time, but should include discussion, current events, art, word games, trivia contests, and music groups.

What you observe should be appropriate to the unit participating in the activity. A discussion of the week's news events on an alert unit would not go very far on a dementia unit. On the other hand, rhythmic guitar and sing-alongs are great on the lower-functioning units; they almost always hold the attention of the residents and magically involve the staff as well. Rosalie Kane, a sociologist and expert on the culture of long-term care, recently delivered the keynote at a medical directors' meeting I attended. She compellingly advised that too many nursing homes offer a plethora of "therapies" as opposed to life itself. Why not call horticulture therapy just plain gardening? The purpose of one's existence in a nursing home should be to continue a real life and not divorce oneself from it.

Trips outside the facility for those who are able are a plus. Volunteers often facilitate the groups but should not be the sole providers of diversion. Activities professionals are indispensable and required by regulation. Though the turnover can be high, these professionals should fairly drip with energy and vitality. Try to meet the activities director if only to get more of a feel for the key personnel. See how flexible he or she would be at working out an individual plan for your parent if needed. Tell the activities director of a particular interest your loved one might have. I once took care of a man who was the first forensic hypnotist in the country. During his career, he had been called in to hypnotize the Boston Strangler in an effort to make him confess! Our activities staff got wind of this and allowed him to hypnotize other residents. It was not only great fun to watch and for the residents to take part in, but it gave him a feeling of identity and worth.

Does the director or therapist appear to possess the imagination to run with a new idea? If there is not a choral group but your parent loves to sing, might they consider starting one? A favorite activity in our home is the New Year's Eve party. We conveniently hold it a few nights before the real thing. The countdown begins at eight P.M. and goes not from ten but from five down to one. Despite that, energy pulsates in the room. Our entire staff helps the residents get ready and dolled up for the big night. The men wear blazers and the women have their hair done in anticipation of the big night. My wife, Lori, our three daughters, and I serve with other volunteers as waiters for the evening. At this point in our lives, it's more enjoyable and moving than any New Year's Eve party to which we could possibly be invited. So ask what they do for New Year's. If the eyes of the staff light up and you can hear the champagne corks popping, it's a sign of a home with a heart.

Family Meetings, Communications, and Councils

As mentioned, the home should schedule a family meeting soon after admission. Usually at about two weeks, the team caring for your family member will have a good idea of how she is progressing and what the near future may bring. If the therapy has gone well this might even be the beginning of the discharge plan. If not, the staff should relate how long they think therapy may take. If your family member is there for antibiotics or wound care, it will likely take even longer and the meeting will serve as an update.

Review discharge ideas. You need to be sure everyone is thinking similarly. As many members of the team should be present as possible but surely the therapists, the head nurse, the social worker, and the activities professional should be in the room. The most important participant, of course, is your parent or family member. The best-laid plans are not worth a hill of beans without the guest of honor in attendance. Be sure that she speaks freely and be sure that *you* share your thoughts, too. You *do* need to put aside your own thoughts after you voice them and listen to the professionals. They will have seen another side of your family member. In the prior few weeks they will have observed her closely and objectively. You also might be able to share your own observations of how she was doing before admission and how she seems to be responding to the nursing home and to the therapy program.

If discharge is in the offing, ask what Medicare, Medigap (secondary insurance), and/or Medicaid will cover for home services. Most people will qualify for some home care for a period of time under Medicare. This can vary from state to state, especially if your family member has Medicaid, too. The services may include a home health aide, physical and/or occupational therapist, social worker, and visiting nurse. The social worker at the home should contact a home health care agency and that agency should contact you to see what you need. The ideal agency sends a representative to the nursing home to evaluate the resident before discharge. In most cases, this is a nurse who can sum up what is covered and what special services or equipment (such as a special bed) are desirable. Homes without much sub-acute care may not remember to call in the home health care agency. If they don't, you should ask them to do so.

The physician will most likely *not* be present at the meeting, but if there are medical issues that are pertinent, it is fair to request that he or she participate or call in. Your chances of achieving this depend on the facility and the physician. If the home has a small, closed medical staff, it is likely that he or she will attend. I do not attend all of these meetings, especially if I have already had substantial contact with the family. However, if the discharge plans depend on medical issues or follow-up is in question, I make it my business to sit in for at least some of the meeting.

Let's look at a possible scenario. If your parent is relatively healthy but suffers a hip fracture, *generally* speaking, by two or three weeks she should be on her feet with a walker and only in mild discomfort. The plan may specify another week of therapy and the social worker will be setting up home therapy and nursing services for a period of time under Medicare. But if therapy has slowed down, it may be due to a number of causes. Perhaps shortness of breath or persistent confusion has prevented aggressive therapy. Your parent may still require complete assistance to get out of bed and two people to help her walk. She may become so fatigued and/or be in so much pain that the slated hour of therapy is terminated after fifteen minutes. The physician needs to be aware of this and act on it.

More often than not, there is a reasonable explanation and the team and doctor can intervene. If the doctor cannot or will not attend the family meeting, then request his or her phone number or have the team contact him and get back to you as soon as possible. Failing that, a call to the administrator of the home to contact the medical director is in order. Assuming they are not one and the same, you might also ask your parent's prior physician to call the present physician. Sometimes that will be enough of a nudge to get a response. Most of the time physicians will want to be involved and be thankful for the questions; it makes their lives easier and gives them a reason to make another visit to your parent. However, there might still be a few hardheaded ones left who need a prod (and I mean a cattle prod). A call from an administrator usually does the trick. The administrator may have heard this several times about the same physician and should get the medical director to act. Perhaps the medical director will switch the care to a new physician if there is not a prompt response or take over the care him or herself. Give the original physician the benefit of the doubt; he or she may have a busy practice or a message may have been missed and they can easily self-correct. If not, be a polite but squeaky wheel. Use that magic phrase, "Wouldn't you do the same if it was your mother?" and really mean it. Advocacy never ends.

Also remember that your family member has significantly changed and has been admitted to the home for a reason. Things are not the same as they were two months or even two weeks ago. The ground has shifted and you need to steady yourself and get your bearings. People age, they fall sick, they become confused, and they need help. If you do not acknowledge these facts, you may do as much disservice to him or her as the doctor who does not return your call or the aide who does not help clean your parent frequently enough.

The team may make recommendations to you that are tough to swallow. For example, the team caring for your parent may have observed what you've been afraid to all along. It may wisely advise that your parent move to the Alzheimer's unit the better to be directed and diverted.

In our nursing home, we currently care for a woman who was brought in by her family about six months ago because they could not care for her any longer. At the time she came in, the family related that she only had a few memory lapses and would be fine on a unit with other alert and conversant residents. When I probed and did a few tests, I discovered that she was also falling frequently, had hurt herself during several of the falls, and that the memory "lapses" represented true memory loss indicative of mid-level Alzheimer's. She was not reliably continent and this had embarrassed and depressed her. To say she quickly became lost on this unit is an understatement. She needed stimulation and direction most of the day and this unit was geared for independent activities, trips, discussion groups, and the like.

The team caring for her met and to a person recommended the Alzheimer's unit as the best unit for her. On the unit, there are directed and highly structured activities. The staff is cross-trained so that the nursing assistants do sing-alongs as well as personal care. In our experience, this would have been the perfect setting for our resident. The family, though, remained and still remains in denial that Mom has a serious problem and in so doing, they are depriving her of a better place to be. It's important to listen to those who are experienced professionals. Acknowledge why your parent is there in the first place and work as a team with the staff. Everyone will be happier...especially your parent.

Try to have an open mind and visit a unit that the team recommends. Though you may disagree, do not tune out its advice. The team members are not there to collude or plot against you; they are professionals who can offer considerable counsel. There may be legitimate safety issues, perhaps your parent needs a unit with more supervision or even locked doors. Create a feeling of collegiality with the team. Use the team meeting to explore the problems and focus on what is best for your parent.

If there is no conclusion as to discharge or placement on a unit, the team will probably request another meeting in two or three more weeks. If not, then *you* should request it. The majority of these meetings end positively and shed light on both sides. Feel free to bring up any care issues you might have as well. If your parent stays for long-term care and does not return home, there should be annual team meetings with you and your parent. You may visit the home often and be satisfied enough to feel that these are superfluous. They usually, however, are a good idea.

Some homes issue report cards quarterly or in advance of an annual meeting. Depending on who fills them out, they may contain incorrect information or may not reflect what you see. More desirable than a report card is the knowledge that you have an open line to anyone at the home and that they respond to your needs as long as they are within reason. A facility is a home, but it is not *your* home. If you could have managed things at *your* home, your family member would not be in the nursing home. As your parent changes, the staff might change or the administration will reorganize or the home may be sold to a new owner. Roll with the punches and be vocal and firm but reasonable in your requests. Be as sagacious as the originator of the Serenity Prayer: "God grant me the serenity to accept the things I cannot change, courage to change the things I can, and the wisdom to know the difference." (And you thought it was from a Hallmark card!) In other words, pick your battles and think today and tomorrow, not yesterday.

Many homes have resident councils with elected officers. These provide a forum at which residents can raise questions directly with the staff. While the discussions sometimes devolve into arguments about how sticky the mashed potatoes are, they as often bring up issues of import. In our state, there is a department of health regulation that staff members not speak foreign languages in the presence of residents. I have some personal issues with this regulation. It has resulted in the placement of Big Brother–type signs that exhort employees to "speak English." However, after attending our home's resident council meeting, I heard firsthand why the residents were so upset when aides or nurses spoke a foreign language. They of course thought that the aides or nurses were talking about them, or worse, poking fun at them. The resident councils enabled me to hear what is important to the residents and we were able to respond appropriately.

The existence of a family council is also a sign that the home is open to ideas and keen on satisfying families. Our council meets several times a year and often sponsors speakers. I have addressed the council several times about issues such as Alzheimer's disease, dementia, flu vaccines, and the like. We had a session recently with our director of pharmacy to explain the problems in the Medicare Part D prescription drug plan. Our family council members even publish a newsletter for residents and their families. The members volunteer at different functions and help set up an annual health fair. It is there that we provide flu vaccines to visitors, hearing tests, and a medical advice booth at which I answer medical questions. To our executive director's credit, he attends the family council meetings and often allocates staff to help implement its ideas.

Getting Caught in the Web?

In looking to review a home, you are likely to go online. While the Internet is a great tool, just beware that the amount of information can be overwhelming. One often can't discern the source of the information. There are some sites, however, that make good places to start and chief among these is the official Medicare/CMS site www.medicare.gov/NHCompare. This site represents a controversial project launched by Medicare to evaluate the quality of nursing homes. The project is known as the Nursing Home Quality Initiative that I mentioned earlier. Remember the MDS (Minimum Data Set)? By dint of the MDS, Medicare has a trove of information on each Medicare-licensed nursing home in the country. One can easily use the site to compare homes in a geographic area.

For example, if you were interested in how a certain home performs in terms of preventing bedsores, you would enter the name of that nursing home. Medicare then compares the home you selected with those in the region, the state, and the country.

The site contains useful information but should not be the sole criterion upon which you base your decision. If the numbers look great, that's wonderful. If the numbers are terrible, ask the admissions director for the most recent state survey report to see if it corroborates the report card. Also ask the admissions director about the report. The prevalence of pressure ulcers may be high but explainable. Perhaps the home specializes in rehabilitation under Medicare Part A and simply accepts numerous patients from a local hospital. Perhaps that hospital does a poor job preventing pressure ulcers and literally transfers the problems that they created—and the mediocre statistics—to the nursing home. Many homes would refuse to care for such residents. To the home in question's credit, its directors of nursing and medicine are willing to take on the challenge.

The official website will also give you useful information such as whether there is a family and/or resident council. You can also evaluate the adequacy of staffing at the home since it lists the number of hours devoted by staff per resident per day. Good homes that are breaking even or are profitable tend to hire more staff since it is the hands-on staff that generally makes a difference in day-to-day care. The flip side is that some for-profit homes may turn their profits over to the owners or shareholders rather than pay for more staff. You should interpret the staffing information from the report with caution since there *are* minimum staffing requirements that the home must meet in order to maintain a license. A well-trained staff with effective leadership and established protocols will accomplish more in less time than a lower-quality home with more staff time per day.

One can also read about the number and types of deficiencies reported during the prior state surveys. It will be difficult to interpret these since they are often worded in generic terms such as "Failed to give each resident care and services to get or keep the highest quality of life possible." It is not clear to me how you would find out what that really means except to ask the home itself or negotiate the state department of health automated operator system. Some deficiencies are very specific and easy to interpret. It *is* worth reviewing this page on the website. If there was a long list of deficiencies, including some causing actual harm, you would want to pause and take a hard look at the place. Sometimes, due to quirks in the survey system, one deficiency compounds into others and the bark of the website is worse than the bite. Most important, though, are the quality measures that compare directly the home in which you are interested to other homes in the area.

Another way to research on the Internet is to search for websites that *help* you compare. Many of these will charge a fee, though usually not more than twenty dollars. I decided to perform a search and found numerous sites but tried www.healthgrades.com. This site evaluates different types of health care facilities, including nursing homes. It can also help you rate a doctor. I was skeptical because it seems to use the same information that is available through the Medicare site.

I requested a comparison of ten nursing homes in my area at which I have either worked or at least visited several times. The review cost me $19.95. The site rates the nursing homes much like hotels, from one star to five stars. I had my own sense of where these homes stood. The ratings matched exactly what I was thinking. The three best homes garnered five-star ratings, while the rest earned fewer stars.

I was encouraged that the local home with a lobby befitting the Waldorf-Astoria, but with a managerial track record like FEMA's

(Federal Emergency Management Agency's), was ranked quite low. Of course, the reviewers on this site never *see* the chandeliers in the lobby. The rankings are based on objective outcome measures. For some, though, the ambience and creature comforts of a place do count. If you relish bright autumnal foliage and the changing of the seasons, then a home with a large solarium peering out into the forest would count for a lot. You might forego the best-ranked home in favor of the one with a view and you might be justified in doing so.

Take time also to analyze the many different quality measures on the Medicare nursing home compare site. The site explains nicely what each measure represents. There are a number of disclaimers that help you interpret and not over interpret the data. Since homes do change (for better or for worse) the data should be updated frequently. Nursing homes are required to submit the quality measures quarterly so the data should accurately reflect the home's current state. If the admissions representative (or word of mouth) tells you that the home has had a dramatic turnaround, ask the representative to explain. The Internet offers some great information, but remember it is merely data. An explanation from the admission representative or someone on staff is essential.

Summary of Chapter 3

- Meet the staff, meet the staff, meet the staff. Besides nurses and therapists, does the ancillary staff (housekeeping, kitchen, reception, etc.) interact with the residents?

- Ask to see a room. Can you imagine your family member in it? Does the tour guide knock before entering and show respect for the residents?

- Are most if not all residents out of bed? If not, can the tour guide or nurse explain why?

- Are activities and groups in evidence? Does the staff engage the residents? Are TVs left on to the detriment of residents? Ask to see the calendar of activities and observe to see if they are posted for all to see.

- Does the food look appetizing and is there off-tray service, linens, etc.? Is there enough staff in evidence to assist residents during mealtime?

- Try to meet the director of nursing and/or an administrator and engage briefly in discussion. For example, you might ask about restraint philosophy or efforts to reduce bedsores. Try to chat with residents.

- Does the home have resident and/or family councils? If they are present, they help to identify the home as a better-quality one.

- Recognize your own gut feeling about the place based on cleanliness, staff demeanor, and conversations with residents. Consider going back to sit in the lobby or walk around a bit. What is your overall reaction?

- What is the home's philosophy on feeding tubes? Ask if you would feel free to follow your loved one's living will if he/she refuses a tube. Is hospice readily available if needed? How many are receiving hospice care? Do residents remain in their own room on hospice (a plus)?

- Is there a formal policy for DNR (Do Not Resuscitate) and/or DNH (Do Not Hospitalize)? Will the home honor prior advance directives or assist you in completing new ones?

▪ Have the Medicare Part D information, vaccination history, and living will ready when you apply.

▪ Fill out the application and strongly consider consulting a competent elder law attorney about assets, Medicaid, etc.

▪ Be sure staff can give you open and honest answers to your questions or refer you to someone who can. The attitude of the staff is key.

4

Transfers and Transitions

The transfer from the hospital (or one's own home) to a nursing home can be as good or as bad as it gets. There are countless opportunities for miscommunication and numerous chances for no communication at all. Needing a nursing home means that the rules of the game have changed; your loved one has entered a different phase, even if only temporarily. It behooves you as a caring person and family member to be sure that all the information that is pertinent is downloaded from the prior situation to the present one—specifically the health information. The social and financial information will fall to you directly, and you will have direct control over that. The medical information is less under your control, but you can go a long way to ensuring its delivery.

Information Download Part I:
From Home to Nursing Home

If your parent is coming from home, which is less likely these days, be sure that the family physician fills out the appropriate forms from the nursing home. Doctors have a great reluctance to complete paperwork. They are swamped with insurance forms, workers' compensation forms, disability forms, and the like. If the doctor has an efficient office manager, he or she may be the best person with whom to speak. The most important form from a medical point of view is the medical history form. There may be a stray nursing home that will not require it. Many homes have enough empty beds these days that they expedite every admission. In these cases, they may go back and obtain the form after the fact or rely on the new doctor at the home to obtain health information. If that *is* the case, it is the rare doctor in a nursing home that will actually call the prior physician. Call it lack of time, sloth, or just bad care, but don't let your loved one be the victim. Be aggressive in pursuing good communication and the transfer of important information.

If the home *has* sent a medical history form, be in touch with the doctor's office to be sure they have received it and are processing it. Often a nurse or manager in the office can simply prepare it for the doctor to review and sign. Sometimes the office will simply copy several recent visit notes, a list of medications, or a recent hospital admission and lab tests. That's great and is often more useful than forms that might be outdated.

You might feel resentful having to handle this since it's the nursing home's responsibility. Some homes have very efficient admissions directors (or social workers) and some do not. Some are just very busy and in a rush to get the person admitted. Don't let it fall to fate. Be aggressive and at least check with the nursing home that they have received the information prior to your parent's admission.

I find it helpful if the family brings in its own list of medications. If that's not possible, then just scoop up all the pill bottles (vitamins, herbs, condiments, and all!) and throw them in a brown paper bag. The doctor may frown but this will provide a real-time snapshot of what's being ingested. There may be so many specialists involved in the care that what the cardiologist prescribed last week may not even have made it to the family doctor's chart. In that case, your own list or brown bag will tell a more complete story than the doctor's notes. Don't get me wrong, the doctor's data is critical because it will list the diagnoses and the reasons that the meds are necessary in the first place.

Vaccination history is important as well, and the forms should include it. The main issue is whether a pneumonia vaccine has ever been received. In most cases, a onetime Pneumovax is sufficient as long as it was given after age sixty-five. More controversial (and experts differ in opinion) is who needs a booster shot after five years. If it was given before age sixty-five or your parent has a history of kidney or liver failure, low immunity, active cancer, or takes long-term steroid medication such as prednisone, then he or she should have a booster five years from the original vaccination. Please check with your doctor. (Some are now recommending a revaccination every ten years.) If such information cannot be obtained or no one really knows, the general rule now is to go ahead and give a pneumonia vaccine anyway. The downside is pretty minimal.

The other important piece of the vaccination puzzle is whether an influenza vaccine has been received. This is especially important during the period from about October to March. Everyone in a nursing home (including staff) should be vaccinated unless they are allergic or refuse. At our nursing home, we also provide vaccinations for family members, but we'll get to that and other infection issues in chapter 11. Most homes will have you or your loved one sign a consent form before receiving either vaccination. If an influenza vaccination was received during the active flu season (fall and winter), it should not be received again. However, accidental or unwitting revaccination is not the worst thing in the world. In fact, certain experts may be recommending revaccination or larger-dose vaccinations in the future (if the national supply can be guaranteed).

Other things that I love to see included in the medical information from a doctor's office are prior laboratory data, such as blood tests, X-rays, and electrocardiograms. These provide a great reference point. For example, most newly admitted residents undergo a basic battery of such tests. It is very common in older people to find abnormalities on such tests. A chest X-ray may show an abnormal left lung that is read as "possible" or "definite" pneumonia. If an X-ray from the doctor's office taken a year ago showed the exact same finding and your parent has no cough or fever or other sign of pneumonia, then he or she does not have pneumonia. The finding on the X-ray likely represents something from the past, and if it shows no sign of change, it does not require treatment. I can't tell you how many such cases *are* treated (most often over the phone with the doctor never examining the resident) with seven to ten days of antibiotics for no reason. This practice exposes the resident to potentially significant side effects and breeds even more resistant germs (bacteria). By ensuring that the doctor is armed with as much information as possible, you can prevent this scenario.

There are other, fancier tests that many elderly have had such as CT scans and MRIs. These are expensive and usually involve time, cost, and transportation. If these tests have been done in the not-too-distant past, there is usually no need to repeat them. By providing records of these, you will save time, money, and the inconvenience to your family member of a trip to a testing center or hospital for a repeat performance. If your family doctor forwards copies of these tests with the records, it is also important they actually go on the chart at the nursing home and do not get buried in an old records section.

I am keen also to see copies of prior consultations with specialists. These are often letters dictated from the specialist to the family doctor. They provide a wealth of information and often prevent the nursing home doctor from duplicating tests and re-creating the wheel. If you happen to have a good relationship with that specialist's office yourself, you might want to get those records directly. It is unlikely that the nursing home will try to contact more than one physician, so the burden may fall on you. If that specialist has not played a key role in caring for your parent, it might not be worth the effort. However, if your parent's main issue has been shortness of breath and a lung doctor has been involved, by all means be sure that the pulmonologist's records make their way to the home.

Don't ignore psychiatrists' and/or psychologists' records either. Those entering nursing homes increasingly suffer from dementia, depression, and even psychosis. Do not be afraid that such care will stigmatize your parent or make the nursing home think twice about admitting them. More than likely the home and physician will find the information helpful in future treatment and avoid retreating with methods or medications that have not helped in the past. If there are severe behavioral issues, such as aggressive behavior or wandering, it is best to disclose these at the get-go. The home will use this to decide on the best level of care within the home. In the rare case that the home feels they cannot manage such behaviors, it is best to know that and find a more appropriate setting. Any home that is gun-shy about even minor behaviorial issues may not be a home that inspires much confidence anyway.

There may be other forms that the nursing home requires for admission from the family physician whether the person is coming from home or directly from the hospital. In general, these will not be your worry since the home cannot proceed without them. For example, some states require documentation that the prospective resident truly needs the care of a nursing home and is dependent in two or three of the six so-called ADLs (activities of daily living) or has significant dementia requiring supervision. This is especially true if the person is on Medicaid and the state is paying the bill for room and board. The powers that be may also require what is known as a PAS (preadmission screening), but again the state will actually send out an official (usually a nurse) to examine and interview the person to be sure nursing home care is necessary. The PAS applies to people either on Medicaid or who may be on Medicaid within the next six months. If there is a primary diagnosis of a serious mental illness excepting dementia (regardless of whether the person is on Medicaid), a PASRR (preadmission screening and resident review) will be needed.

The need for a PAS and/or PASRR can cause a logjam since the Medicaid office usually has only a few nurses who perform them. If a person is to be admitted to a nursing home for sub-acute care and a PAS cannot be arranged, the hospital prepares a transfer sheet signed by a physician that states the patient is approved for twenty days or less. If the patient later proves to need long-term care, the nursing home will request a PAS. In New Jersey, the Medicaid office is required to send a nurse within thirty days but check your state for local requirements.

Information Download Part II: From Hospital to Nursing Home

The more common situation occurs when the hospital directly transfers your parent from the hospital for short-term rehabilitation or for long-term care. In this case, there may still be requests from the doctor's office and that's fine; every bit of information helps. The more important data here is what arrives directly from the hospital. Since your parent was sick enough to be admitted to the hospital, the treatment plan and medications will more than likely have changed. The hospital is motivated to proceed with discharge and in most cases will have faxed preliminary hospital records to the nursing home. The receiving facility will then have an inkling about the incoming person. It will be able to judge if it can provide care and what special equipment might be needed. It might also reject the person. Some of these decisions are related to clinical reasons, such as the need for a private room to contain resistant infectious bacteria. Some considerations are due to cost. Remember, if your parent is under a short-term Part A stay, the nursing home receives a fixed amount of money from Medicare per day. The discharging physician might have prescribed two exorbitantly expensive antibiotics and a special wound treatment that together cost more than Medicare reimburses the nursing home. The for-profit homes will in many cases refuse to admit these people. What the homes sometimes don't realize is that the treatment may be able to be tailored to something more reasonable *and* with equivalent clinical results. In lieu of this, the home could say it will accept the person in transfer after the antibiotics run their course. The home has a fair amount of leverage in these scenarios. While no home wants to sit with empty beds, it may be hard-pressed to accept a peron who will, before adding in the costs of nursing care and food, be a losing proposition. The hospital may fish around for another facility but often will be stuck eating the costs of care. This is only one of many reasons why hospitals are mostly in the red right now.

The records that are faxed are only preliminary and should certainly not be used for the final list of medications. While they *may* be current, they probably are several days old and medications can change hourly in a busy hospital. The reason this is so important is that you want to be sure that your loved one gets the *correct* medications when starting out at the nursing home. You need to be aggressive in making sure this happens. One fail-safe you can ensure is that on the day before *or* the actual day of transfer, ask for your own copy of the medications and orders from the hospital and bring them over to the nursing home yourself. You will then be able to engage the physician in discussion or, more likely, have the nurse at the home go over the lists to make sure they jibe.

Do not accept a common parry by nurses that HIPAA (Health Insurance Portability and Accountability Act of 1996) laws prevent them from disclosing protected information. HIPAA was created to prevent insurance companies from denying coverage to people with preexisting conditions. Secondarily, it was intended to secure personal health information. This means that personal information should not be read by people to whom the patient would object reading it. The law did not seek to deny concerned family members the right to know how their loved one was doing. In 2004, the *Washington Post* reported an egregious case of a family that was not notified by a certain hospital that their missing loved one was killed in a car accident because it feared a HIPAA violation. The family found out he had died several weeks later when it received a bill for his care. How the hospital had the correct *billing* address but claimed no permitted contact information was unclear.

The New York Times carried an illustrative story in its July 3, 2007, edition. Nurses in an emergency room in Illinois told one Gerard Nussbaum that he could not have access to his father-in-law's medical record and invoked the HIPAA law. Little did they know that Mr. Nussbaum was a health care and HIPAA consultant; he did not take the news lying down. The law states that health care workers *may* share health information unless the patient demurs. Misinterpretations of HIPAA give too much leeway to the health care worker and the path of least resistance is to say "no information." Disclosure, according to *The Times* article, is voluntary, but the patient can designate in writing or dictate verbally who is allowed access to private information. If you have a power of attorney or guardianship, it should suffice. Therefore, with regard to medications, do everyone a favor and try to get a copy of the medications.

In the best of all worlds, this should not be necessary. Every hospital has a transfer form or "inter-facility transfer form," which should contain all vital information. *Should* is the operative word here. The rub is that many hospitals seem unable to compel the doctors to fill out the forms. In my medical community (and I see these forms by the dozens as we accept residents in transfer to the nursing home), some hospitals are able to get their physicians to fill out the forms and some are not. To cut them some slack, the discharge often coalesces at the last moment—the doctor might have office hours all day and not be able to get to the hospital. But, really, there is no excuse. I'm no technocrat, but isn't that what fax machines are for? Go figure. What it boils down to (in my humble opinion) is that some hospital cultures simply don't place the patient first.

Some hospitals get around this by simply copying a computerized list of medications and attaching it to the discharge sheet. Unfortunately, these lists can be several days old and not reflect the up-to-date list of medications. Moreover, due to glitches in hospital computer systems, some key medications are listed as treatments as opposed to medications and get left off the printout entirely. My local hospital finally realized that a medication called Coumadin (warfarin) was one of these omitted medications. This is a very tricky medication that thins the blood and is used to prevent blood clots and strokes. The reason that it is so tricky is that the wrong dose (or no dose) can spell disaster. The hospital finally changed the computer entry for this medication, but only after about a year of complaints (from yours truly...forget blood *thinning*, think blood *boiling*!). And while I'm ranting, wound treatments and breathing treatments are often listed separately as well and never make it from the hospital to the nursing home. The bottom line is that if the doctor doesn't fill out the form, there's really no guarantee that everything's up-to-date.

Even if the doctor fills out the form, he or she may omit key information. Nursing homes often admit patients who have just undergone hip replacement or hip fracture surgery. Much of the time, the most crucial information is missing from the transfer sheet and that is whether the person can bear weight on the affected leg. As my kids would say, "What's up with that?" There is a range of different fractures and operations and each might have different orders for weight bearing. Given the disappointing lack of information, I often need to comb through the hospital chart (if the hospital sent a copy), call the orthopedic surgeon, or let the physical therapist try to ferret it out. In most cases, we do arrive at a coherent and correct plan, but why should it be so hard and take so much time?

One would think that after all those years of medical school and the requisite training, there would be some pride in making sure that the good care delivered in hospitals would not go to waste. In my twenty years of taking hundreds if not thousands of people in transfer from hospitals, I have been called perhaps five times by a physician to discuss a transfer (and all those were doctor friends of mine who knew I was on the receiving end). Medicare, state review boards, and the American Medical Directors Association are looking at this, which can only be good news.

I hope this verifies the importance of "moving day." You can do a great service to your loved one by facilitating information transfer. Try also to supply the nursing home doctor with a list of prior doctors and their phone numbers and be sure the information finds its way into the nursing home chart. I try to call the family on the first day or two after the move. I usually have a few questions about prior care and/or medications. I also want to home in on the prior functional status of the person. Two people with the exact same list of diseases and medications can be quite different in terms of their ability to get up and around and take care of themselves. If the goal is short-term rehab to return the person home in a few weeks, then I like to know what we're aiming for. The therapists handle the nitty-gritty on this front and perform a detailed assessment, but I like to know what the big picture is. Admittedly, since I work in the nursing home, I have the luxury of being able to contact the families a little more easily. However, the majority of the times, I *can* speak face-to-face with family members on the day of admission, since they often accompany the new resident to the home. If there's a chance that by waiting another hour or so, you will have the chance to meet the doctor, I think it's well worth it. You will facilitate further communication and get a good sense of what issues might arise in the home.

If your mom or dad is supposed to be on oxygen, be sure they continue it at the home. If they're not supposed to be on oxygen, then ask why they're on it! You should also have an advance directive or living will available *or*, in lieu of that, at least know what your loved one would say. Clearly, if he/she is alert and with it, then they can communicate that to the physician directly. See the discussion on living wills in the last chapter of this book.

Other Things to Think About: Making It Homey

There are many non-health-related issues to deal with on transfer and those are best handled by prior discussion with the home's admissions director or social worker. For example, is there a "patient's needs" account that provides ready cash for things like haircuts, trips, special meals, etc.? Do you need to bring in several changes of clothes? Who does the laundry? Is there a television or telephone in the room and, if not, how does one hook up service? Some of our younger residents have been bringing their own cell phones and that might not be a bad idea. Are valuables safe? Even the best homes have some problems with theft so don't bring expensive jewelry, diamond rings, etc. Crime can occur anywhere and the temptation is sometimes just too great.

One other piece of advice: Bring in pictures and personal effects that make people want to stop in the room and chat. One or two favorite pieces of furniture (if the home allows) really make the room look homey. Recent or long-ago family pictures on the walls help orient the resident and provide them with a sense of comfort. I love seeing a one-hundred-year-old's baby picture above her on the wall. Sometimes the face and expression are so utterly the same that one can only gasp. If your loved one painted, bring in a painting or two. The family of the aforementioned forensic hypnotist brought in an article about him. It lay on a table next to his bed and always made for great conversation. A woman for whom I cared until she died at 102 had a particularly intriguing picture on her wall. It showed her at her sweet sixteen party dressed in a harem outfit reclining on a divan with a cigarette dangling from her lipsticked mouth. I suppose at that time (1918), anything Ottoman was the rage! It was still the rage at our home, and on holidays and at open houses people would come to see her *and* the picture. She also could recite multiple stanzas from Tom Lehrer songs on demand. Now *that's* entertainment. So gussy up the place, make it a trophy room of sorts, and invite the world to come in and make friends with an individual who has earned a place to call her own.

Summary of Chapter 4

- Be sure your loved one's doctor completes the medical forms from the nursing home or sends appropriate records including specialist reports.

- If coming from home, bring a complete list of medications or put all medications in a bag and bring them with you.

- If coming from the hospital, be sure accurate and up-to-date transfer sheet and medication list are sent or fax/bring it yourself. See that therapy orders are written if applicable.

- You may need to be the general contractor for the transition. Advocate!

- PAS (preadmission screening) may be needed for long-term care, especially if Medicaid is paying.

- Do not be put off by a claim that obtaining information violates HIPAA rules.

- Be sure the hospital discontinues intravenous lines, urinary catheters, and other appliances if not needed in the nursing home. Clarify if oxygen is still needed or not.

- Make the new room as homey as you can. Bring photos, books, mementos, and personal touches.

Part II

Navigating the System

5

Dramatis Personae: A Personnel Scorecard

While not exactly a cast of thousands, there are several key personnel that make a nursing home run. Let's go in order of who you and your loved one will meet. Before we go down that path, though, please consider that working for the elderly may not be for everyone and working with the frailest institutionalized elderly is *certainly* not for everyone. There are some special people who work in these environs, and describing some of the scenes I have observed has filled me with emotion and my eyes with tears. As the saying goes, though, one bad apple can spoil the whole bunch. There have been and will always be bad apples in nursing homes as in all walks of life. Don't let them distort your view of the industry.

In conversation, I often hear about how insensitive or incompetent a particular nurse's aide was. I acknowledge the disappointment but quickly cite cases of the many saints with whom I have worked. Denigrating a whole class of workers over the actions of a few becomes self-fulfilling: They will never measure up. But if you give the workers the benefit of the doubt and treat them politely and with respect when they slip up, *you* will be happier and *they* will provide better care. Don't forget that nursing assistants, in particular, often work below a living wage, often in pain, doing messy and draining work. The clients they clothe, feed, medicate, shower, and try to love sometimes spit at them, kick them, and bite them. The clients also sometimes call them the nastiest names in the book, but the staff cannot react or they might be fired. Think about how long you would survive working in roles like these.

The nursing home business is said to be the second most regulated in the United States. (The first is the production of nuclear energy and waste!) A nurse or social worker these days can expect to spend at least one-third or more of his or her time on paperwork. Some of this time is spent writing on the patient's chart, but much of it is filling out the countless forms that regulations say must be done. Each time the government advances a new regulation, whose beneficent aim is to *improve* care, it generates more paper and steals more time from face-to-face care. While administrative work is a necessary evil, next time you're upset that staff doesn't seem as admirable as you'd like them to be, remember that nursing home employees are required to do so much that takes them away from direct care.

Director of Admissions

The first person you are likely to meet in a nursing home is the director of admissions, though the director is usually the only admissions worker there is. He or she is often a social worker, but need not be. The admissions office, not unlike a college admissions office, is there in part to give you a good first impression. It is best suited to someone with a wide and genuine smile who can process and keep track of many details. The admissions director also helps to decide what nursing unit or section of the home is best for your loved one. The director will often consult with the nursing home team, including the nurse, social worker, and sometimes the physician. This placement is sometimes done subjectively; a few homes have more objective "placement tests." It is best for everyone that your parent be admitted to the correct unit in terms of cognitive (mental) function as well as physical needs. Different units have different numbers of staff and a higher-functioning unit may only use a skeletal staff at night. You will not be doing your parent any favors by holding out for one of these units if she needs a lot of physical care. The activities on the unit are also geared to the average person on the unit. I sometimes see residents with advanced dementia struggling to keep up with a discussion group on current events. Usually this is someone we had recommended for a move to another unit but the family resisted. I understand the resistance; who would want one's loved one to move in with more debilitated and less verbal residents? But it is truly for his or her benefit. The frustration at having to keep up causes anxiety, agitation, or worse. So don't impugn the staff with any ulterior motives. Many homes will actually have you sign a form at the get-go that gives them the right (which they already have) to move a resident if the resident needs more care.

The larger the home, the more variety and the more exact the placement. At our home, we have six units based on the different permutations of physical and cognitive abilities, and we staff them differently. This helps us distribute the labor pool fairly. If a person with Alzheimer's has a major problem with wandering, we may need to at least start him on a locked unit—i.e., a unit where the doors are locked and staff can only get in or out with a code.

No placement is perfect; some are based only on available rooms. If you do not like a placement, say so and ask for an explanation.

If the admissions worker admits that only logistical problems necessitate such a placement, ask to be on a waiting list for the next available room. Private rooms, by the way, almost always cost extra, though if it is needed for infection reasons, most facilities will not charge.

Sometimes a placement is a mistake. Sally was a favorite resident of mine. She developed a severe pneumonia while living at home. Her physical abilities were already compromised before she fell ill and she had no close family around. When she went to the hospital, she was delirious due to high fever and low oxygen levels. This improved considerably, but her hospital records were laced with the words "dementia" and even "probable Alzheimer's." No one had taken the trouble to investigate her prior mental function. Since we have a terrific dementia unit, we placed her there. From the moment she arrived on the unit, *she* knew something was wrong. When she asked around and realized where she was, she told anyone who would listen that she didn't have Alzheimer's. I guess it's a credit to our place that people eventually took her seriously and moved her to our highest-functioning unit, but it took several days to happen. Her experience may not be so common but it reminds us to always give the benefit of the doubt to the patient.

The Staff Nurse

After the admissions director moves your parent to her assigned unit, the next person you're likely to meet is the staff nurse. Each unit has one or more nurses assigned to it depending on the number of residents. A typical high-functioning unit in our building has fifty residents and we have three nurses on the day shift, two on evening, and one at night. This is far less coverage than in an

acute care hospital where ratios are about eight patients to one
nurse, depending on the unit, of course. Then again, nursing home
nurses don't need to make beds and clear a lot of bedpans. In nursing homes, that work is done mainly by nursing assistants. The
nurses spend most of their time handing out meds. They also perform wound treatments, relate to families, answer countless phone
calls, leave countless phone messages for countless doctors who
can be hard to reach, supervise the nursing assistants, break up
disagreements between residents, follow every regulation in terms
of documentation, complete the Minimum Data Set in a timely
way, and so on. With whatever time is left, they are expected to go
to more and more training/educational sessions and smile as much
as possible. You can see that it's a thankless job and I can't imagine
pulling all that off. But without nurses there would be no *nursing*
homes. The nurses really are central to the culture and success of
any home.

Nurses come in at least two different types: the LPN (licensed
practical nurse) and the RN (registered nurse). RNs have more
education and have completed more course work than LPNs. They
also have more training in assessment than LPNs. An RN must
supervise LPNs in a nursing home. In many ways, though, the LPNs
perform similar work to the RNs. They both pass out medications,
change and clean wounds, administer breathing treatments, and
complete documentation regarding their residents. They each can
evaluate a resident who is short of breath or experiencing chest
pain. All things being equal, you would probably like to see a home
with more RNs on duty, but in many homes it is hard to find or
afford RNs. Many homes have mostly LPNs, and an RN nursing
supervisor or manager is present for oversight.

More important is the experience the nurse has had and in what
other settings the nurse has worked. Many RNs have worked in

acute care hospitals and are comfortable around sick patients. This can cut both ways. Certainly a resident with significant breathing issues who may need suctioning from a congested windpipe will benefit from a nurse who has worked on a respiratory unit of the hospital. The nursing home, however, is *not* the intensive care unit and a nurse with an acute care mentality will sometimes overdo it. For example, I had a patient several years ago who every single day complained of chest pain and claimed she was dying. We had performed the appropriate electrocardiograms and other tests for chest pain. She even underwent a modified stress test that determined that her complaints were not related to her heart as much as to anxieties about dying. An RN with a very aggressive ICU attitude might have missed the point and called 911 for the emergency rescue squad. What the resident needed was someone to sit down and talk to her about her worries. So I ask you not to judge a book by its cover. Some LPNs with years of experience in a particular home may be top-notch.

Finding enough quality nurses is a major issue and begs a discussion of agency nurses and foreign-born nurses. Agency nurses are provided by an agency ad hoc to fill in holes in the schedule. The nurses move around to different homes and rarely stay in the same place for long. While agency nurses may be lovely people and good nurses, they often do not know the residents of a home well. They don't know how each one prefers to take her medications or how each resident behaves day in and day out. And if they are not familiar with the residents, then all the king's horses and all the king's men can't put the nursing home together again. A disconcerting image is watching an agency nurse look in her medication book at a photo of a resident to be sure she's passing the medication to the right patient. Our home has been fortunate never to use agency nurses, but we are the exception.

Due to the shortage of nurses and relatively low wages in some facilities, many homes employ foreign nurses. There are regional trends but this is the reality in almost every part of the United States. I can't imagine where we would be without nurses from overseas. Some are sponsored by the host facility expressly to work here and many have had to pay fees to immigration lawyers to enable them to remain. In our home, we have nurses from the Philippines, Ghana, Liberia, Senegal, Kenya, Nigeria, Barbados, Jamaica, Grenada, Guyana, Haiti, Bulgaria, Russia, India, Sri Lanka, and Korea. It certainly brings wonderful exotic aromas to our staff lunchroom. My own experience has been excellent, but there are issues that arise. One is communication. As fluent as these nurses often are in English, they sometimes have thick accents that are hard for residents and/or staff to understand. Heavily accented English spoken to someone with hearing and other sensory deficits may as well be a different language.

This is not meant to denigrate these foreign nurses. Those I've worked with have been professional, compassionate, and highly qualified. But I mention the possibility of potential communication problems so you can get an accurate picture of what is happening in long-term care today, and so that you can be vigilant and make sure your loved one isn't experiencing any problems communicating with those who care for her.

Upon admission, a nurse performs an assessment and completes some more paperwork, then he or she will do a body check. A body check is akin to checking out a rental car before you drive it. Both the rental agency and client agree that the car was in a certain condition (dings and all) at time zero. The body check serves to document in what condition the resident's skin is on arrival. The nurse carefully notes any skin breaks or sores or old scars. The most likely person to help the nurse do the assessment and help transfer the person into a bed is the certified nursing assistant or CNA (also called nurse's aides or orderlies).

The Nursing Assistant

The CNA is in just about every way the backbone of the long-term care facility. She or he is the most underrated member of the team, but the one who knows the resident the best. Whenever I want to know how a resident is doing—for example, if he is eating normally or thinking coherently—I ask the CNA. Most CNAs in most facilities follow and care for the same group of people each day and they know them better than the families do. While I have heard my share of comments about how lazy some CNAs are or how they "just sit around," I am in constant awe of how they do their work and lead their lives with dignity and grace. They often relate to the residents with respect and care. I have seen plenty of CNAs cry when a resident dies and have driven several to funerals. I have seen them stoop to rearrange jewelry and reapply lipstick or replace a religious article that may have dropped from a resident's hands. What is more amazing to me is they do this while being grossly underpaid and being verbally and physically abused by some residents. Due to dementia, residents often lose the ability to filter their feelings and aggression. I have treated many CNAs who have been bitten, scratched, kicked, punched, fondled, and spat at. I have heard the epithets and the profanities heaved like bombs from demented or just plain bigoted minds. How the CNAs do their jobs without lashing out is beyond me; their self-restraint is remarkable. They often have health issues, financial, and personal problems galore. When you have a chance, read *Nickel and Dimed: On (Not) Getting by in America* by Barbara Ehrenreich.

The author goes undercover and tries to survive on a series of low-wage jobs. The most poignant vignette to me was when she became a nursing assistant in a nursing home. Reading it might make you think twice the next time you criticize a CNA.

The CNA provides what is known as personal care. This includes getting the resident out of bed, washing or showering him, taking the resident to the toilet many times a day (or changing adult diapers), escorting him to the dining room, placing a tray of food in front of him and/or feeding him, changing his undergarments when they get soiled, wheeling or walking him to an activity, and then reversing the dressing and toileting when the resident goes to sleep at night.

Each CNA has between six to eight residents to take care of for the average eight-hour shift. Start doing the math and you can see how exhausting a regimen this is. It's kind of like taking care of septuplets, each weighing over 120 pounds and each with an attitude! The getting in and out of bed or in and out of the wheelchair means physically lifting a good deal of deadweight if the resident cannot assist you in your efforts. Some can assist, but many cannot. Now you know why some assistants may want to take a breather and sit down on a well-deserved break. You and I would want to do the same.

The training for a CNA is significant, but depends on the state. A high school degree or its equivalent is sometimes required as well as training in first aid and/or CPR. The certification process involves a certain number of hours of training in a state-approved program. The federal Nursing Home Reform Act of 1987 mandated that nursing assistants receive at least seventy-five hours of training and some states require more. They must then, according to the AARP website, pass a certification test within four months of commencing work at a nursing home. In addition, they must receive at least twelve hours of continuing education each year. At most facilities, they receive more. Several advocacy groups have recommended a higher standard of up to 100–120 hours of training. Such a commitment might cut down on the high turnover rate experienced by many facilities.

Besides the tasks outlined above, the CNA also takes vital signs, cleans dentures and brushes teeth, cleans and makes the bed, gathers soiled linen and laundry, and makes entries into the chart or care plan.

The care plan is a key concept and is what ultimately drives the day-to-day care. The plan itself is written down and is kept on the unit; the CNAs and nurses refer to it often. Care plans are highly individual and should reflect the particulars of taking care of a human being. The basic personal care details are written but also any dietary likes and dislikes, how to feed the resident, how they like to be bathed, what to do if they become agitated, how to respond to abusive behavior toward the staff, and what time they go to bed...just for starters.

The Nurse Manager and the Nursing Supervisor

Now let's go up the chain of command. In the nursing hierarchy, some homes will have a nurse manager or charge nurse, who not only performs nursing functions but also manages the nurses and aides. Because he or she manages all three shifts, this is a great responsibility and not for the faint of heart. The nurse should have good communication skills, get the big picture, and be able to respond calmly and honestly to a resident's and family's questions or complaints. The charge nurse will often be the liaison between the staff on the unit and the administration and be present at some of the committee meetings in the home. The extent to which this happens is a function of the home. The more the home seeks to empower the staff, the more likely the nurses and aides will be asked to be present at such meetings. For the sake of everyone's well-being (residents and workers), a staff whose feelings and observations count will be more responsive and creative in its own work. Nursing homes have been slow to embrace this model, but it is gaining traction. We can't afford *not* to bring the aides in to help us make decisions. They know the residents better than anyone.

The nurse manager or charge nurse also has a major responsibility to make sure the MDS documents are accurate and that the individualized plan of care reflects them. When opportunities arise to improve care, this nurse often will enlist the help of the family or doctor or activities therapist to effect the change. The unit nurse manager is the quarterback of the care team.

The next nurse to consider is the nursing supervisor, who is akin to a town crier, roaming the alleyways of the home even at the crack of dawn to announce all is well. The supervisor changes with each shift (standard shifts are morning, afternoon/evening, and overnight). They help coordinate the schedule and plug any holes that might arise. This is easier said than done; there are always absences, illnesses, and vacations. The supervisor also interacts with outside services such as hospitals, ambulances, labs, doctors' offices, and radiology suites. They might help a nursing unit that has three new residents and that is busy completing paperwork make sure that all established residents have received their medications. They are often enlisted to work on special seasonal projects like giving out influenza vaccines or routine issues like infection control. Our night supervisor periodically makes the rounds to every bed in the home to make sure the chart orders for bed rails being in use are accurately reflected in the rooms themselves. There are few things worse than a resident falling out of bed and breaking a hip because a bed rail was down that should have been up (which is by no means to say that all bed rails should be up).

On nights and weekends, the supervisor functions like an administrator since he or she is the top staff person in the home after hours. Families, as they say, "don't know from weekends" and rightfully expect answers to their questions at all times. The supervisor must be able to represent the home intelligently and honestly and are drawn in many different directions. One of our supervisors even trapped an overly inquisitive raccoon in a Hefty bag and delivered it to animal control. How's that for being a team player! The supervisor can be your best friend: When you call or have a problem over a weekend that the staff nurse can't handle, all roads will lead to the supervisor. So treat them with respect and I think you'll find they'll try to help you out. They tend to be the most experienced and smartest of the lot. Even when you call the home after hours, the supervisor usually functions as the switchboard operator and has a finger on the pulse of the building.

The Director of Nursing

The director of nursing (DON) has arguably the toughest job in the whole shooting match. The DON does not have direct hands-on nursing responsibility for any one resident, but in a sense is accountable for the care provided to all. The DON has an idea, along with the supervisor, of when a resident "just doesn't look good." She should be present at any meeting that affects the residents and delivery of care. For example, at our home a partial list of committees includes wounds, falls, corporate compliance, infection control, quality control, pharmacy and therapeutics, and for good measure we threw in a dining committee to upgrade the dining experience. The DON becomes stretched pretty thin with all this, and she often sits in on family meetings, budget, construction, and planning groups to boot. She will often help the admissions director look at hospital records to see if the home can care for a resident.

The DON is ultimately responsible for work schedules for the nurses and nursing assistants. This seems to be the single most challenging and angst-inducing task. It is very hard to find good and capable nurses who will work all kinds of hours and stay long enough for the orientation and training to have been worth it.

The DON also shares responsibility for investigation of accused abuse. Under recent legislation, the reporting laws on abuse in long-term care are very strict. For example, in New Jersey, any suspected case of abuse must be reported to the state ombudsman's office. This includes resident-to-resident abuse with injury, which—because of the large numbers of residents with dementia—happens not infrequently. Suffice it to say for now that the DON has a lot on his or her plate. A good administrator can help unload some of this, particularly some of the committee and abuse work, but when you call the DON for a question, you might not get a callback quickly. It makes more sense to start with the nurses on the floor and see if you can't get some satisfaction that way. Some homes also have an assistant DON (ADON) that can really serve the same role and may be more available.

Either the DON or the ADON may be a good route to the physician if you are having trouble getting in touch. Of course, this depends on their working relationship and how amenable the physician is to answering questions. And by the way, most states have chapters of NADONA, the National Association of Directors of

Nursing Administration. I recently had a phone conversation with its national director. I can tell you she gets it and has a wonderful vision of the potential of long-term care in this country. She and NADONA are advocates for nurses to be sure. Check out their website if you have time or have more questions about the role of long-term care nursing (www.nadona.org).

The Therapists

If your parent is at a home for short-stay therapy (sub-acute or Medicare Part A), she will receive an early visit from the therapist. This might be the physical therapist (PT) or the occupational therapist (OT). The head of the therapy department in our facility happens to be an OT. Sometimes he is the first to see a new resident and assesses exactly what regimen of therapy will help restore the greatest amount of function. For example, if your parent just had a stroke and has trouble moving both the right arm and the right leg, she will almost certainly need the help of both the OT and the PT. As a general rule of thumb, the OT works with the arms and the PT works with the legs. Occupational therapy is really a term that harkens back to a time when a disabled worker received therapy to help him return to his prior occupation. These days, most rehabilitation candidates are not returning to an occupation per se. The goal is to return them to their prior level of function. Now *that's* a tall order especially when there's been a loss of mental sharpness from a stroke or dementia. In the best of all worlds, though, that's what it's all about... getting people back into their best potential physical and mental shape.

I regard a good therapist as worth his or her weight in gold, and for short-term residents, the bond with the therapist is often

the "make it or break it" of the experience. The majority of therapists are hardworking, energetic, dedicated, honest people who
love what they do and derive great satisfaction from their work.
They often point out medical symptoms that might need attention.
I try to visit my patients during therapy to get a sense of their progress. When things don't go well, it is worth asking if any therapy
sessions were canceled and why. Medicare mandates a certain
number of hours of therapy per week in order for the home to be
reimbursed. The home has a great interest in seeing that this happens and I rarely see a therapist at fault. Know that the reporting
of hours to Medicare is an honor system (if and until a home is
audited). While I have never seen it happen, an unscrupulous home
could shortchange hours or keep someone on rehab who no longer
benefits from it.

More likely is the scenario that the resident declines therapy.
Perhaps she is still too exhausted from the hospital stay and illness to participate. A good therapist will try again later in the day
or the next day when the resident feels more energetic. Perhaps
the resident is in too much pain. Shoulder, hip, spine, and pelvic
fractures are notorious for causing pain that impedes therapy. A
good therapist will be in touch with the nurse or physician quickly
to suggest well-timed and appropriate medication to alleviate the
problem. A dose of a painkiller one hour before therapy may be all
that is needed to set the therapy in motion once again.

The resident may also have motivation problems due to depression or anxiety and these could be alleviated with interventions
by a social worker or psychologist. Medications are available as
well, though antidepressants often take up to a month or more to
be effective. Ritalin, which is used for attention deficit disorder in
the young, *can* be used as a jump-starting antidepressant in the
elderly. If the attending physician is not familiar with its use, sug-

gest a psychiatrist to consider prescribing it. Studies have demonstrated its relative safety even in cardiac patients in whom it was once feared.

Another looming issue for failure of therapy is confusion on the part of the resident. In order to progress in therapy, one needs to build each day on principles learned the day before—like a fourth-grader learns math skills. Division builds on multiplication, which in turns depends on the foundations of addition and subtraction. If the student can't absorb and retain the fundamentals of addition, there is little chance of succeeding with advanced math functions. So it is with therapy. If your parent has problems with short-term memory and can't remember the skills from the therapy session the day before, there is little chance that therapy will advance the cause. One also can distinguish between mild confusion and severe confusion or early Alzheimer's and advanced Alzheimer's. The former conditions should allow for therapy while the latter often will not.

Even with mild confusion, the resident may absorb enough from therapy to improve, albeit slowly. A good therapist here can be a godsend since he or she may have tricks to help teach a client who is confused and suffers memory loss to retain new information. I once cared for a ninety-something-year-old who broke her hip in a fall. She had moderate Alzheimer's, thought the year was 1940, and that FDR was president. I swore there was no way she would learn to walk again. Owing to the motivating skill of our über-therapist, she not only walked but fairly sauntered. As if to prove it wasn't a fluke, half a year later she broke the other hip and sure enough became mobile again after surgery.

Recently I was walking the halls of our home and saw a woman walking next to a physical therapist. When I drew closer, I nearly fainted at recognizing her. This was a very old woman who had come to us about two months prior and had been shriveled up in bed in a fetal position. I would have wagered that she would not walk again, much less survive. And here she was walking, chatting, and smiling! So sometimes, as they say, ya never know!

Confusion that starts in the hospital may not be related to dementia as much as to delirium—a more temporary form of confusion that many of you have encountered with family members. The physician will likely pursue treatment of the delirium. Our friend the Minimum Data Set assessment tool is particularly good at picking up on delirium, and nurses have sometimes notified me of a new delirium based on the MDS assessment protocols. The physician should attempt to isolate the cause of the delirium and treat it if possible. Favorite remedies are removing medications with side effects, improving the oxygen levels of a resident, or merely waiting for the tincture of time to heal it since most delirium clears by itself. If confusion persists, or the resident has entrenched dementia, such as Alzheimer's, the therapy program may not proceed successfully.

And now back to the different therapists and the kind of therapy you will encounter. OT involves not only the arms and fine motor skills, but also the overall ability to complete or execute tasks. (This is sometimes known as *executive function*.) Eating, or rather feeding oneself, is a great example. A stroke affecting the right side in someone who was right-handed compromises the ability to use utensils to feed oneself properly. Therapy might involve improving the strength of the right side and/or teaching the person to use the left side more. There is a plethora of silverware devices and special plates that can greatly assist. The OTs are masters at this. In addition, a change in the consistency of the diet to food that is softer and doesn't need cutting can help the person eat independently.

The OT also helps the PT in transfers. Transferring, in rehab speak, means the ability to get from one spot to another. What we take for granted—such as getting up from a chair or getting to the toilet when we want to—represents a Herculean task for some residents. Some of the work has to do with equipment like sliding boards or removable arms on a wheelchair, but much of it involves cognitive sequencing of a task. Just as you teach your teenager what the sequence is for pulling out of your driveway (check mirrors, foot on brake, gear shift in reverse, turn and look, etc.), an OT can teach someone in rehab how to get from the bed to the chair. The therapist breaks down the task into a sequence of mini-tasks and can understand whether the person's cognitive abilities suffice. Sometimes repetition and cues can help. Most of the time the OT must work as a team with the PT. The smoothly functioning body is not just about the arms *or* the legs, but is a symphony of many different parts conducted by the functioning parts of the mind.

When not directly collaborating with the OT, the PT coaches people who need to walk again after a hip fracture, hip replacement, a knee replacement, or even prolonged bed rest. The range of procedures on these joints is large and growing, and each has its own peculiarities in terms of how much weight one can bear on each leg and when it is safe to do so. I will discuss hip fractures in chapter 7, but the PT is a great person with whom to stay in touch to chart progress. The PT should be in periodic contact with the orthopedic surgeon to determine when a patient can graduate from walker to cane to being free range again. The PT also should have ready access, at least through notes and messages, to the attending physician if there are pain issues or concerns about mental changes, which are quite common.

PTs and OTs are experts in nonmedication modalities to control pain. They utilize deep, moist heat massage; hot paraffin baths; ultrasound; hot packs; cold packs; even old corn husks to decrease pain and increase mobility in arthritic joints and healing bones. They generally need a physician's order, but I have not heard of too many physicians who have been uncooperative. The treatments become part of the comprehensive plan of therapy and at times can spare the use of heavier medication. If you wish to ask about non-traditional methods of pain treatment such as acupuncture, you should feel free to ask, but I would wait until you see if the standard therapies fail. If your parent is someone who has benefited from alternative treatments before, then I might press the issue earlier. Medicare does not cover acupuncture, though some private insurance partially pays for it. For an excellent source of information, visit www.nccam.nih.gov, the website for the National Center for Complementary and Alternative Medicine.

The therapists will sometimes bring in a speech therapist for one of two reasons. After a stroke affecting the left side of the brain, there can be neurological damage that results in trouble finding, understanding, or speaking words. This can range from partial loss or dysphasia to complete loss or aphasia. The classification of these is difficult and depends on where in the brain the stroke took place. (There can also be slurring of words or faulty articulation known as dysarthria, which happens in strokes of either side.) The other major reason to call in speech therapy is if there is trouble swallowing properly. Dysphagia can be the result of Parkinson's disease, stroke, Lou Gehrig's disease, or most commonly Alzheimer's disease. The speech therapist, though usually not in the home full-time, performs diagnostics at the bedside by watching the resident eat and drink a variety of different-textured foods. Based on this he or she might recommend a certain diet or therapy sessions to teach the resident the best way to eat despite the disability (see chapter 12 on feeding tubes and nutrition). *Occasionally* the therapist will recommend a modified barium swallow test, which is a fancy set of X-rays looking at the mechanics of swallowing. This will always involve a short same-day trip out of the nursing home. It is particularly useful if the person has developed an aspiration pneumonia (food going down the wrong pipe into the lungs) or sounds like she is coughing, choking, or gurgling after eating. While most speech therapists are reasonable, some are overly zealous and write in the chart that the resident should have nothing by mouth (NPO). See chapter 12, but know that these recommendations can put you and the team in the awkward position of considering an artificial feeding tube that might be against the resident's specific wishes as expressed verbally or in a living will. Be strong and don't let the therapist's recommendations rule the day. As a group, they are beginning to come around, but in my opinion, slowly.

There should be at least one family meeting about halfway through the course of therapy to review the progress and to begin talking about possible discharge. The resident, if she is at all able, should attend since the team will advise on some major decisions. If therapy has gone well, the team will begin to assess what kind of help or further therapy can occur at home. If the therapy has not gone well, each member of the team and the family needs to be creative to determine the best options. Certain families will have the financial resources to provide enough care at home despite the lack of return to independence. A visiting nurse service should consult to determine what Medicare or other private insurances will provide at home. Many long-term care insurance companies cover at-home expenses as well as facility costs (it's cheaper for them in the long run). Sometimes the therapists can actually visit the home and advise on any modifications that need to be made, such as a grab bar in the bathroom or a glider up the steps. They can also check for safety snags such as throw rugs and electrical cords.

The ability to view the therapy sessions during a short-term stay is particularly valuable. When residents make swift gains, the family begins to trust and value the facility and the therapist(s) and can begin to plan for the homecoming appropriately. On the other hand, when your family member's therapy is slow, you need to ask whether it is due to a problem with the therapy and nursing home or with your loved one. Finally, get over the idea that only the doctor (unless possibly it is a physical medicine doctor, aka *physiatrist*) can tell you whether someone can go safely home. The medical problems and list of medications are *usually* not the make it or break it and the doctor has no monopoly on seeing into the future. The PT and OT will have the best sense of whether a discharge home is feasible or safe and what human and/or mechanical aides need to be in place for the plan to succeed. So learn to love and trust your therapist. If you were stranded on the proverbial desert island and wanted the best chance of surviving, bring a therapist with you...you won't regret it!

The Social Worker

At some point soon, you will meet the social worker, which may or may not have been the admissions director that you already met. The general social worker assigned to your parent functions almost like a guidance counselor in school...they both look out for the general welfare of their charges. She or he is also a good place to start with any troubleshooting. Don't be too hung up on titles. Many homes have youngish bachelor's- or master's-prepared social workers while a few have licensed clinical social workers who can and do perform psychotherapy at the home. It really depends on the market in that area and also to what extent they can be mentored and supervised.

The social worker helps take care of everyday life for the resident. While each home's division of labor is somewhat different, most social workers see to financial issues such as social security payments, applying for Medicaid, deciding on whether the room and nursing unit are appropriate, and whether roommates and tablemates are good matches. If a unit is the wrong unit, they work (and work and work!) with the families to effect that change. The social worker should also schedule and coordinate family meetings. More than that, their skills should enable them to decide when family meetings are important. Some family meetings are mandatory as when a discharge plan is being assembled. Other family meetings are called when families have problems that the regular staff does not seem able to solve.

Most family meetings are useful and I think they impress on the family that the staff is made up of professionals who work together and know their residents well. The family also needs to hear that the resident is *not* the same person she was three months ago. If she were, she would not be living in a nursing home. I take the attitude that with every complaint there is at least a grain of truth. Some families are dysfunctional and bring that into the home. Social workers are adept at setting ground rules so that the family dysfunction doesn't spill over into the home. Sometimes we need to involve the individuals' lawyers but most families will agree to disagree in order to help Mom or Dad.

The social worker is an advocate for the resident. If the resident complains that a physician or nurse is not listening or that an aide is rough in terms of physical care, the social worker needs to begin to find solutions or someone else to whom to refer. The family, as an extension of the resident who may not be able to express himself, may make similar requests and I sometimes receive calls from the social worker telling me that a family is concerned over a change in mental abilities or behavior. The social worker, or anyone for that matter, may suggest a psychiatrist or psychologist if the primary physician seems unable or unwilling to intervene; often the medical director needs to assist in these situations and has the power to do so. In our facility, the social worker is the liaison to the psychologist since he or she can relate the particulars of a case. Many social workers also perform more mundane tasks, such as seeing that dentures, hearing aids, and glasses are in working order or are being ordered and repaired. They also sometimes chart and track missing items. With all that, and being relatively underpaid, this is a discipline with high burnout.

The Activities Therapist

The activities therapist will at some point wander into the room to do an activities assessment. These folks can be the life of the party. Once a year, I give a lecture to our state society of activities professionals and it's always quite a ride! They have nonstop energy. One website advertising a certification program for activities professionals described them as focusing on what is *right* rather than what is wrong with their clients.

You might be wondering exactly what an activities professional does. (They are still sometimes known as leisure or recreational therapists, too.) Well, let's put it this way: Even if a home provided perfect nursing, medical, and social work care and had Wolfgang Puck running the kitchen, its residents would waste away from boredom without keeping busy and enjoying themselves. There *are* the few residents these days who prefer to entertain themselves by reading, watching movies, and playing solitaire, but they are going the way of the quaint "rest home." It remains to be seen if the boomers of the near future will be such cyber-fanatics that they may be content pushing a mouse and tickling a keyboard in the privacy of their own room. By and large, though, residents in nursing homes need things to do, and the activities professionals provide these diversions.

The key to a good activities program is akin to the success of differentiated learning in primary schools. Nursing homes support residents with widely divergent mental abilities. Some nursing units may have a preponderance of alert and coherent residents and others have very few. Almost all floors are mixed to one degree or another. The bulk of the activities that occur on the unit should be geared to the common denominators and not the outliers. Smaller groups, one-on-ones, or activities off the floor can cater to different needs.

As with social workers, different homes staff differently. The market is a bit tight right now and activities *assistants* are easier to come by and don't cost as much to hire. Our director made the decision to use more assistants and has found that they go a longer way. You certainly get more coverage in terms of ratio of staff to residents. With the changing face of long-term care and the increasing number of people with dementia, this is a good thing.

Some activities groups I have witnessed in recent years appear to have been dumbed down. Contrast this to an activities professional I witnessed when I was in training in the mideighties who led a slide show for residents displaying different themes in European Impressionist art. He was excellent and able to draw in staff and residents alike. I'm afraid that kind of program may be all but extinct. Then again, it's case by case and professional by professional and maybe somewhere it still exists. The danger of a not-very-good program is allowing it to degenerate into babysitting and bingo. Creative activities professionals often have a specialty in art or music and are much sought after.

In any event, the activities professional performs a thorough assessment and describes how that resident likes to spend her time. There is usually a question or two about religious and/or spiritual interests. The activities team often coordinates religious services as well. There will always be residents who cannot be dragged out of their rooms for anything. What you must understand, and we get this all the time from families, is that we cannot force someone out of her room or make him sit through an activity against his will. Some families *can* help if they are actually present and reinforce it. Some activities staff is better at cajoling than others, but the reality is it only has so much time and may have fifty other residents to transport to a concert room. If it's any consolation, the feds actually use as a quality marker what percentage of residents does not participate in any activities. The state and federal survey (and now the public, too, thanks to report cards) teams have this data and will zero in on it during inspection week if it's out of kilter.

The Dietician

The parade continues and next we present the dietician (or nutritionist at some facilities). No one is dispassionate about food at a nursing home. There are individuals at our own home who feel each meal should be a culinary masterpiece, though I doubt that reflects their prior eighty years of dining experiences. I have stayed at my own nursing home overnight on several occasions and eaten the residents' food. While I am not the most discerning gourmand,

I found the food tasty, varied, and wholesome. But try telling that to the residents. The role of the dietician then is to try to bring some objectivity to this whole messy topic and, above all, to match the taste to the diet. The dietician aims to satisfy these needs while keeping the intake as healthy and medically appropriate as possible. The intake assessment should explore medical requirements such as diabetes, blood pressure, and salt intake; evidence of malnutrition and weight loss; possible kidney or liver disease and protein intake; and history of problems swallowing (dysphagia) or holding utensils (apraxia). That's the easy part. The hard part is the taste issue. While to each his own taste has a basic appeal, it really cannot be satisfied in all homes. The dietician works hard to match the taste buds to the other competing needs of the resident.

If the resident has an inordinate fondness for lamb chops but can only swallow a soft or pureed diet, he or she might be up the creek without a paddle. There are some high-end alternatives such as "formed" meals, for example, in which lamb meat is pureed and then remolded in the form of a look-alike lamb chop. This cost is usually out of the reach for many homes, but might work for tiny places, if restricted to the Alzheimer's unit, or even for one resident once in a while. For all the piss and vinegar I've heard about food all these years, I'll never forget a resident named Sadie. She led a very tough life in public housing in lower New York City. Several men abandoned her along the way and her kids developed severe mental illnesses. When we admitted her to the home, she immediately gained twenty pounds and told us she had never had it so good. And the best part…the food! So I do take the food complaints with a grain of salt. I've seen dieticians work very hard with residents and families to satisfy their likes and dislikes. The dietician also may help with diet waivers that allow the resident or family to make informed choices ignoring so-called medical diets. He or she will usually confer with the physician first, but ultimately should be comfortable in pursuing a waiver.

If there are questions about diet, weight loss, chewing habits, mealtimes, supplements, meal partners, and/or overly restrictive diets, the best place to start is with the dietician. Some are hip and understand that the resident is in his or her own home. If at home a diabetic can raid the icebox (as my residents still call it) at midnight and eat key lime pie with butterscotch sauce, they need to have the same rights at the nursing home. Other dieticians are less aware and will not easily bend. In those cases, it's worth going to another branch of the service, such as the administrator, for a second look.

The Administrator

And speaking of the administrator, this is where the buck stops. Each home has at least one administrator, who is a licensed nursing home administrator (LNHA). Some LNHAs come to it from a business background, some were destined from birth to do it, some arrive via family connections, and some just fall into it. The administrators at our home are involved in almost every aspect of the home as well they should be. There is rarely a meeting that does not include at least one of them. It is their license that is on the line should bad things happen. They are answerable for any issue that affects the home and they coordinate the formation of all policies and procedures. They ensure that we are staffed adequately, they create and balance the budget, and they interact with the state and federal agencies at survey or surprise inspection time.

The administrator often appropriately delegates work to others. When the state ombudsman receives a complaint about care or possible abuse, he or she will call the administrator, who then will most likely refer it to the director of nursing to investigate and meet with the state official. If a family complains about a certain doctor, the administrator will seek out the medical director to research the case. Needless to say, a strong medical director, or supporting staff for that matter, makes the administrator's life easier. Administrators in for-profit homes turn over more frequently than in not-for-profits. Many for-profit homes, at least in the Northeast, are part of a group of nursing homes usually owned by the same person or family. In other areas, there are mega-chains as typified by Genesis, Beverly, Mariner, and the like. My experience is that administrators in these homes move around as the need or owner requires. There is always a home in the group that needs more direction or whose finances need shoring up, and the seasoned administrator transfers over as a caretaker. My own home is indeed fortunate to have had one chief administrator for the better part of thirty years. His two assistants have tenures approaching ten years. This provides extraordinary stability to the home. They know our families and our community and our staff, and it is reflected in our low employee turnover rate.

You should interact with the administrator when you feel you are not able to solve an issue with one of the clinical staff directly. Let's say as an example that your loved one is not out of bed early enough in the morning and whenever you visit she is soiled. You have addressed it with the nurse and/or nurse manager on that floor. You come back next visit and it's déjà vu. You could very well go to the director of nursing or the director of social work, but you choose the former. You palaver a bit; she is gracious and deems this unacceptable, which is great to hear from a DON. You think you've got it licked, but on the next visit it's the same old thing. You're starting to feel like Sisyphus. I would then write down as many of the details as you can and request a meeting with the administrator. Spell out exactly to whom you have already sent the problem and make it clear the response was not adequate. If you have time, compose a quick letter; that always seems to attract attention. You needn't make any threats at this time, but if you are stymied or ignored, then you might make mention that the state department of health or ombudsman's office will be hearing from you soon. The administrator may only recommend a family meeting with the staff and the social worker, but that often is the right setting to begin solving festering problems. All most people want is a seat at the table. They know one can't make an older person young again, but they want to be respected and listened to. Staff often gets so caught up in being defensive that they lose sight of how useful a family meeting can be.

While some LNHAs are sympathetic and entered the field for the right reasons, don't necessarily expect the warm and fuzzies. They are under tremendous pressure on all fronts, and their purview, which is the entire home, is larger than anyone else's. They do have an interest in providing good care and that will be the ace up your sleeve. Good care means good reputation means more referrals means full beds. So be positive and look to the LNHA to help you move forward in getting the best care for your parent. If anyone gets the big picture, it is the LNHA.

The Pharmacy

Before we get to the medical team, be aware that pharmacy issues are best handled with the pharmacy itself. Most homes use special pharmacies that service nursing homes exclusively and know their business well. The pharmacy bills can be outrageous if you pay privately (as opposed to being on Medicaid). What has tempered the run-up in the bill has been the advent of Medicare Part D, the once notorious prescription drug plan. I say notorious advisedly since from your parent's point of view this plan will save a lot of money. The plans have placed the burden mostly on the facility, the doctors, and the pharmacies themselves. Many of the problems seem to be smoothing over. There are still medications not paid for, holes in the coverage, and confusing bills. The nursing home should refer you to its account manager from the pharmacy, which will be the most direct way to glean information. In a similar vein, you should direct questions about the bill from the nursing home to the business office. There should be a person within those walls who knows what is being billed and can explain it to you in human terms. If not, then seek out the administrator.

The Medical Director and the Attending Physician (Including NPs and PAs)

The medical director represents an administrator of another sort. Many of the nursing home reform rules that the government generated in 1987 stemmed from shoddy medical care that pervaded nursing homes. The regulations legitimized the role of the medical director. The idea was to have a place where the medical buck stopped. A nursing home could no longer throw its hands up in surrender. It could no longer use as an excuse that the home did not employ the physicians and had no control over their behavior much less their competence. The raison d'être of the medical director *is* to supervise the physicians and ensure good care. But let's talk about the attending physician before coming back to the medical director.

As I stated in chapter 2, the attending physician is the doctor assigned to take care of your parent. The nursing home may assign the prior community doctor that role, though often the community physician does not perform nursing home work. In this case, the home will then assign your parent to someone else. This is the proper person with whom to communicate about medical care, medications, continuity issues from the hospital, changes in condition, follow-up visits with other doctors, and whether discharge is medically feasible. On that score, it is always worth keeping an open line with the therapy team that may have more insight into the physical aspects of living at home.

Many nursing home physicians are fly-by-night in the sense that nursing home work is a sideline and they spend 90% of their time in the office or the hospital. They may make rounds (i.e., see the patients at the facilities) at seven A.M. or as late as nine P.M. and you will likely never meet him or her during the course of a regular day. You might want to check with the nurse to determine the best time to find the attending physician at the home. If they happen to make rounds during the normal lunchtime, it might make it easier for you. I personally find it easy to call the family right after I see the resident for the first time; there usually is some piece of data missing or a phone number of a specialist I might need. I also want to introduce myself and let them know how best to reach me. Remember, I work exclusively in long-term care and the majority of my time is spent at one home so I have the luxury of being in touch.

There are a growing number of homes that are subscribing to the medical staff model whereby a few motivated and knowledgeable physicians each take care of a large number of residents. This ensures that they are present almost every day. Since the homes in this model employ the doctors, they also have more control over their practice and behavior. Most of these homes tend to be in big cities or are state- and county-run facilities. The bigger faith-based homes also seem to have adopted this model. But even absent this framework, the medical director should be able to fill the void.

Getting a doctor to call you back can be an exercise in frustration. You might try telling the person who answers the phone that it's urgent or you need a call back *today or tomorrow at the latest*. Another way is to leave your name and number with the nurse or DON to give to the doctor the next time he or she is at the home.

In most states, the official mandated time to visit a new patient in a nursing home is within the first week of admission, but most facilities require a visit within the first forty-eight hours and for good reason. The resident, especially after coming out of the hospital, is often sick and needs attention. The medications need to be ordered over the phone immediately on arrival and it is foolhardy to approve these medications without examining the records and the patients first. After that, the official requirement is every thirty days for the first three months and then every sixty days after that. In practice, though, most nursing home doctors expect to see their patients once a month for routine examinations. If someone is sick or develops a fever, the doctor needs to be notified right away by the nursing staff. The doctor then decides if he or she needs to physically go in to make a visit. They might order the nurse to take vital signs every eight hours for two days, draw a blood count in the morning, and plan to evaluate on their next visit in a few days. They may make a practice of only going to the home once a month to do the routine exams and handle everything else over the phone. Too often, some of these physicians use the local emergency room to handle these "emergencies" and have the resident shipped out in the dark of night to a cold and crowded place. The ERs become resentful, often physically restrain the resident, and place a urinary catheter in them whether they need it or not. It's just bad practice and in my opinion way too common. There are alternatives to this approach that I discuss below.

If the doctor is not responding at all *or* if the doctor *does* respond but doesn't seem to get it, you can try a few things. You can talk to the social worker or the administrator to see if the squeaky wheel gets the grease. Don't be unpleasant or cranky but be direct and say things like you "only have one mother" or "wouldn't you do the same if it was your mother?" The powers that be may be able to get the doctor to be more responsive, but don't count on it. The medical director should be the one to intervene next. The role was created exactly for this reason, so try to exploit it. If he or she cannot seem to get traction with the physician, some medical directors overrule the attending and write appropriate orders or examine the patient anew.

You do have an ace up your sleeve and that's part of the resident's bill of rights. You have the right to a physician of your choice, which you can interpret to mean you can switch to another physician. The ability to switch doctors assumes that another physician will be willing to take on the role. Some are gun-shy when they hear there's been a problem and assume it's a difficult family. Others are glad to pitch in and do not much care what anyone else thinks. Oftentimes, the medical director will be willing to fill that role. Sometimes they don't need to take over officially but just ride shotgun for a while until things straighten out. That's what I prefer to do. In some homes with the staff model, there is one doctor per geographical unit of the home. Switching doctors means violating the integrity of this structure and really isn't a good idea. Luckily, most of these homes have a medical director who is willing to shadow the physician until the problem is resolved.

That said, there are situations in which the family is not realistic and the attending physician *is* acting responsibly. The reassurance of the medical director should be comforting. There are also peculiar personalities in my field as in all fields. I once supervised a very skilled geriatrician who just rubbed some families the wrong way. A family meeting with the doctor present was usually the ticket to get everyone working together. Don't feel trapped or angry, but use the good offices of the home to reach a tenable compromise. The last (and I mean last) card to play is to call the state ombudsman's office from the department of health. We will talk more about this later.

While the medical director should be the ultimate arbiter of medical care issues, there has been a growing trend to use other health professionals to improve care and communications. The so-called "mid-level" practitioners are the nurse practitioners (NPs) and physician's assistants (PAs). I would say the former are much more common in long-term care than the latter and some states have regulations that make it easier to use the NP in this role. NPs have a nursing degree and extra clinical training that qualifies them as an "advanced practice nurse." In most states, they can function very similarly to the physician, but they need to have a collaborating agreement with a physician. This is a document that defines what kind of treatment plans they both agree to and how they will communicate with each other. In some settings (mostly rural or in public facilities) the NPs are highly independent and use the physician for backup if a resident is acutely ill or needs to be hospitalized. At present, the routine monthly visits can alternate between NP and doctor so the doctor will see the resident at least six times per year. The physician must make the first visit and do a complete history and physical exam. Some (few) homes and practices skirt this requirement so it is worth asking if a physician actually saw and examined your newly admitted loved one.

Because of the lack of access by nursing homes to physicians in many areas of the country, these regulations are under scrutiny and my guess is that we will see fewer restrictions on the mid-levels as time marches on.

Usually a physician group or large facility hires NPs and PAs and they are very accountable to their employers. This is a major advantage already. You will find the mid-levels more accessible, more communicative, and having more time than the average physician. They should be able to meet you at the home or at your parent's bedside to review the care and even go over the medical chart and orders if you wish to review them. But, you may ask, what about quality? How could a nurse practitioner possibly have the experience and knowledge of a physician who spent countless hours training and caring for complex patients? Well, I'm glad you asked. Let's put it this way: Long-term care is not quantum physics. It requires a careful eye and a good heart and knowledge of basic medicine. Moreover, it takes someone with an interest and training in the geriatric syndromes that most physicians either never learned or in which they have no interest. When I trained as an intern and resident, a lot of my time was spent with patients in intensive care or cardiac care units. I learned how to manage machines and fancy catheter lines as much as I learned anything else. Much of what I learned I have never needed since I finished residency. So all that extra training and those diplomas that look great don't always provide an edge in long-term care.

I have worked with many mid-levels over the years and I am often astounded by their abilities. On top of that, if I can generalize, they are nurses who want to improve themselves educationally and professionally. They tend to be go-getters and communicate well. Many are certified in geriatrics (GNP-C, where "C" stands for certified, though some are certified in family medicine). They are familiar with issues like falls, incontinence, osteoporosis, dementia, and cognitive changes and know more about nursing home regulations than the majority of physicians. Suffice it to say that the NP or PA is usually value-added and you should view it that way. Of course there are some lemons in every bunch, so if you feel that the mid-level is not measuring up and you can't get access to the physician, go through the same chain of command as I discussed above.

There are several innovative insurance programs around the country that are using a collaborative model between physicians and nurse practitioners to advance the care in nursing homes. The largest and most successful of these is known as Evercare and I will discuss it later in chapter 9 since you may encounter it along the way.

The State Ombudsman

Now that wraps up the cast of characters in a nursing home. However, if all else fails you can contact your state ombudsman's office. The ombudsman is an advocate for older people who live in nursing homes and other long-term care settings. I would not overplay this card and I certainly would not use it as an idle threat. However, the Older Americans Act mandated the creation of a program for each state because some homes were not policing themselves properly. Most state programs are similar. The California office summarizes its role as "to investigate and endeavor to resolve complaints made by, or on behalf of, individual residents in long-term care facilities." These complaints may be of abuse and neglect, but can be related to general care issues, too.

The ombudsman's office may or may not be able to help you if you need to take it that far. It may try to intervene over the phone, but we (and all nursing homes) have been visited by volunteers and staff from the department for specific complaints. These days, this is just part of doing business. Many volunteers actually circulate in the homes to which they are assigned and troubleshoot so as to avoid a crisis from developing. Each state office's number can be found by calling the Administration on Aging's national Eldercare Locator at 1-800- 677-1116 (or visit www.eldercare.gov/Eldercare/Public/Home.asp). Another way to access information is through the National Citizen's Coalition for Nursing Home Reform or visit www.nccnhr.org. I would try to work things out with the staff of the home first, but if you can't or if you feel your loved one is in jeopardy, call the ombudsman. Some homes will frankly hold it against you, though they cannot retaliate in any meaningful way. It *can* cause awkwardness in your relationship with the home, so be judicious.

6

Medications: Just Say No?

Nancy Reagan, when not consulting astrologists to help bolster her husband's political fortunes, busied herself as an antidrug crusader. To some, her advice to "just say no" belied her understanding of the problem. In the realm of long-term care and geriatrics, though, her advice strikes a chord and "no" means "no" to trolling drug companies, begging family members, and doctors more than willing to add a prescription to the pile and move on to the next patient. We live in a drug culture and it affects society's aged as much as it affects our adolescents. The theme of this chapter could be summed up as "less is more." One of my favorite medical cartoons shows one patient whispering to another in the waiting room, "I've never felt so good since I stopped taking those pills the doctor prescribed."

Paper Bags and OBRA

A gaping hole in the quality of long-term care before nursing home reform was the use of medications. Geriatricians coined the term "polypharmacy" to describe the overuse of medications in the elderly. In the outpatient realm, polypharmacy means different things. Sometimes one practitioner prescribes without knowing what another practitioner already prescribed. Even a well-meaning physician can duplicate medications or classes of medications.

When I worked as a primary-care geriatrician we performed the so-called paper bag test. We asked new patients to bring in all the medications they currently were taking in a brown paper bag. This was quite informative as some would haul in a veritable shopping bag full of meds. What was interesting was that they often were taking redundant drugs, such as Advil and Aleve (both from the same family of anti-inflammatory drugs and both potentially causing stomach ulcers and/or kidney problems).

Polypharmacy can also mean a doctor prescribing a medication to undo the negative side effects of a previously prescribed drug. For example, a commonly prescribed medication called Haldol can cause symptoms similar to Parkinson's disease. Instead of stopping the medication or changing to another, a second medication such as Sinemet, which treats Parkinson's, is added. The list of medications grows inexorably and reproduces itself like the sorcerer's apprentice.

Sometimes the patient is partly at fault since he or she refuses to leave a physician's office without a new prescription. Much of the time, the physician simply doesn't have the time to research carefully enough what the patient is already taking. The physician follows the path of least resistance and prescribes something to placate the patient. The potential for side effects, especially in the frail elderly who are more prone to toxicity, is great. Similar things happen in the nursing home and the OBRA regulations seek to protect the residents from this dangerous practice. OBRA refers to the Omnibus Budget Reconciliation Act of 1987 and is the moniker by which the Nursing Home Reform Act is known.

So how to do it? A recurrent theme in OBRA was the lack of trust the feds placed in the system; this included the physicians who prescribed the medications. OBRA '87 required that a "consultant pharmacist" review each resident's medications once per month for several quality issues. In order that there would be no conflict of interest, the consultant had to be independent of the pharmacy that dispensed the drugs. The consultant was to review the medication to be sure that there was a proper diagnosis for which the drug was given, that the dosage was appropriate for the elderly resident, that monitoring of side effects and blood tests was done, and that the drugs were weaned if they should be. This culminated eventually in the "Beers List" of medications (after Dr. Mark Beers who compiled the list), which is a kind of Santa Claus's list of which drugs were naughty or nice. The list is controversial, but serves as a good starting point to limit the use of medications that are particularly nettlesome in the elderly. The newest iteration of the state surveys of nursing homes, based on federal guidelines known as F-tags, is explicit about the dangers of medications. It firmly establishes when and how doctors need to wean certain medications and greatly decreases the wiggle room that practitioners exploit to avoid making these changes.

It takes two to tango and the doctor should not be labeled the only bad guy in the mix. He or she often prescribes medications at the request of families. The anti-Alzheimer's medications such as Aricept and Namenda are great examples. These medications show very little *functional* benefit in the frail, institutionalized elderly and yet families often insist on them. They are uncomfortable with the idea of "doing nothing." Nurses, on the other hand, are on the front lines and are bothered more by the symptoms that residents with dementia evince, such as aggression, screaming, banging, kicking, wandering, and biting. They frequently call the physician and ask for a quick fix. That usually means prescribing medications like sedatives and antipsychotics. All of these have potential side effects such as drowsiness, falls, and confusion. Nevertheless, when used specifically for psychotic symptoms (paranoia, hallucinations, and delusions), the antipsychotics can be helpful.

Sometimes the nurse (or doctor for that matter) needs to be educated in the theory of unmet needs, which is to say that many behaviors are rooted in hidden physical needs of the body. For example, severe constipation will upset anyone, especially a resident with dementia who cannot express herself and whose abdomen is becoming more distended by the day. The unmet need is the ability to move her bowels and doing so will sometimes relieve the agitation. Even if this is truer in theory than in practice, it behooves the care team to explore all possibilities. In fact, geriatrics as a discipline distinguishes itself from the rest of medicine in exactly this exercise. A good geriatric assessment or examination pays special detail to physical aspects of the body that might manifest themselves as symptoms of dementia.

Let's look at several classes of medications that doctors commonly prescribe for nursing home residents. Rather than go name by name or medication by medication, a look at groups of drugs gives us a better handle on types of problems. While there used to be one or two medications per class of compounds, today they proliferate and it is virtually impossible to keep all the names straight.

Antihypertensives

Medications that combat high blood pressure are commonly prescribed in nursing homes. While we used to think that the elderly needed a higher blood pressure to keep blood flowing to the brain, we now accept the fact that the lower the pressure the better...but only to a point. And that's the rub. At what juncture does one try to peel away some of the medications? Certainly when the systolic pressure (top number) begins to go below 110, I worry that at other times, like after eating, it may dip to dangerous levels well below 100. At those stages, there is diminished blood flow to the brain and other vital organs and the result is a fainting spell or "syncope."

There is a phenomenon known as post-prandial hypotension, which was elucidated by a mentor from my geriatric fellowship days, Dr. Lewis Lipsitz. Dr. Lipsitz is a fine researcher and his genius was in following nursing home residents and monitoring their blood pressure as they went about their daily lives. He found great fluctuations in blood pressure and profound dips after eating. It was also at mealtime that the residents received most of their medications. The double whammy of medications *and* meals both reduce blood pressure and put the resident at risk of fainting. The resident might not be able to tell you she felt "woozy" or "light-headed" and then fainted. The staff observes it only as a fall and by the time it checks the blood pressure several minutes later, it returns to normal.

If your parent looks weak, isn't focusing, or does not seem as sharp as usual, it's worth asking about blood pressure. Since a nursing home is not a hospital, the nurses do not check blood pressure as often. In sub-acute residents who have been discharged from the hospital, the staff checks the vital signs more frequently. If your loved one is in physical therapy, the therapist will sometimes check the blood pressure during the sessions, but don't count on it. A low blood oxygen level can also cause a similar picture without the resident recognizing that she is short of breath. Most homes have a small portable machine called a pulse oximeter, which attaches to a fingertip and registers the blood oxygen level. If the level is much below 92%, it may indicate a shortage of oxygen to the brain and vital organs and the staff should notify the physician or nurse practitioner at once. There are a few caveats to this. The machines can be unreliable due to low battery power and difficulty in picking up an adequate pulse, which is how it measures oxygen in the first place. A "normal" level of oxygen is good news. If the number is low, the staff should move the clip that goes over the fingertip to another finger and wait a good few minutes. Certain few people simply will not register a reliable number but a persistently low number *is* cause for concern. In this case, the nurse should obtain an immediate order from the practitioner to administer oxygen.

Again, it is your right to see and review the list of medications with the nurse or physician. The families of medications that reduce blood pressure are the beta-blockers, calcium-channel blockers, angiotensin-converting enzyme inhibitors (ACE inhibitors), angiotensin-receptor blockers (ARBs), diuretics (water pills), and drugs that work on the nervous system such as clonidine. If the staff is not helpful, you can certainly ask for the names of any blood pressure medications and ask your pharmacist or check it out online. There are a few other medications that while not specifically antihypertensives can cause a drop in blood pressure. The anti-Parkinsonian medications like carbidopa-levodopa (Sinemet) and some of the antipsychotics often used in demented residents immediately come to mind.

Other Cardiac Medications and Blood Thinners

Amiodarone (Cordarone) is a medication that has been around for many years. Recently cardiologists have begun to prescribe it to the frail elderly. Amiodarone is representative of the antiarrhythmic class of medicines. Antiarrhythmics regularize abnormal heart rhythms. Amiodarone is officially FDA approved only for life-threatening ventricular arrhythmias, the more unusual and lethal type. The caution owes to the toxicity that this medication can cause. The more common use, and this is entirely off-label as far as the FDA goes, is for a common arrhythmia called atrial fibrillation. Many elderly suffer from this condition, which is also known as AF. The top half of the heart (the atrium as opposed to the ventricle) contains a natural pacemaker embedded in the heart muscle tissue. As the heart ages, damage accumulates and the normal pacemaker rhythm goes a bit haywire.

The dangers of atrial fibrillation are several. The heart can beat much too quickly and therefore less efficiently and this compromises the pumping action of the heart. Much like a piston in a car that doesn't have time to fill with gas and oxygen, the heart simply is not clicking on all cylinders. Restoring a normal rhythm can improve the function of the heart. The question is at what price?

The problem with amiodarone and its cousin drugs like sotalol (Betapace) is that they have pro-arrhythmic effects. Paradoxically, they can in about 3–4% of cases cause more serious arrhythmias than they are designed to abort. Amiodarone also is a hard-luck drug in that it can cause thyroid disease and in 10–15% of people potentially serious lung problems. This is not a drug that amateurs should prescribe. Antiarrhythmics should mostly be started by a cardiologist and in a hospital with a cardiac rhythm monitor in place. Did I mention they can also cause inflammation of the liver? Another kicker is that amiodarone lasts a long time and may take a month to clean out of the system. If side effects develop, your body is stuck with it for weeks! Now, all that said, if a resident of mine has rapid atrial fibrillation that is compromising her overall function and it *can't* be controlled with other medications, I'm open to trying amiodarone. However, I would want to be sure that at a certain point the drug has achieved its desired effect and converted the person's heart rhythm to what we call normal sinus rhythm. Absent that conversion, I would speak to the cardiologist about stopping it.

There are many cardiologists and other experts that, based on recent studies, say that amiodarone is a lot of malarkey and don't advocate its use. If one simply controls the rate of the AF and combats the stroke risk (see below) with a blood thinner, adding amiodarone does not improve quality of life, much less survival. For a fuller discussion of this, please see the Atrial Fibrillation website at www.a-fib.com. Suffice it to say that far too many frail elderly are placed on these toxic medications. If someone prescribes an antiarrhythmic for your loved one, ask questions and try to understand from the cardiologist why it was started and whether it's working.

In lieu of amiodarone, medications that physicians use to modify the rate of atrial fibrillation include the beta-blocker group, the calcium-channel blockers, and a centuries-old medication called digoxin (Lanoxin). The last of these is held not to be as effective, but is still commonly used. The beta-blockers like Lopressor, Toprol, and atenolol (Tenormin) and the calcium-channel blockers like diltiazem (Cardizem) and verapamil (Calan) can simultaneously treat hypertension and angina. That provides synergy and can be a smart approach if both of those conditions are present.

Another risk of atrial fibrillation is an increase in strokes. Because blood tends to pool in the top half of the heart during atrial fibrillation, blood clots are more likely to form. These clots can travel up to the brain and cause a stroke. Many studies have shown that well-monitored use of a blood thinner called warfarin (Coumadin) can protect against strokes. All things being equal, atrial fibrillation equates to the use of warfarin. But things are never equal when it comes to frail and elderly denizens of nursing homes. The studies that demonstrated the utility of warfarin certainly did not include nursing home residents. The risk/benefit ratio of warfarin narrows in this population. What you have to understand is that warfarin is a kind of poison; it actually is still used as a mouse and rat poison. It thins the blood by paralyzing the natural clotting system of the body. A little too much warfarin, and the blood won't clot at all. Internal bleeding can be the result. Moreover, if an older person has any tendency to fall, a simple knock on the head can cause massive bleeding in the brain and spell disaster. This can happen even if the warfarin is monitored closely. I am loath to use it on anyone who has fallen or looks like they might fall. There are others whose intake and compliance with medications is so erratic that one can't hope for a steady level of the medication.

The commonly used blood test to monitor Coumadin is the PT/ INR, also known as Pro-Time or simply INR. For most people with atrial fibrillation, the INR should be between two and three and should be measured at least once a month. If the medical team needs to adjust the dose, the level should be repeated in a few days. Warfarin can cause extensive damage in nursing home residents, no matter the good intentions of its prescribers. If the team deems the risk/benefit ratio as unfavorable, a simple aspirin once a day can serve as a poor man's warfarin. Most studies show partial protection and it's a lot safer.

Warfarin is also used in other scenarios. Blood clots in the legs and lungs (deep-vein thrombosis and pulmonary emboli, respectively) must be treated with warfarin usually after a few days of injections with medicines like heparin or enoxaparin (Lovenox). Warfarin takes several days to thin the blood, hence the need for the other medications in tandem. The treatment lasts ideally for six months. If bleeding complicates the treatment or the person is too high risk for a blood thinner from the get-go, one alternative is a filter or "umbrella" device, which a surgeon or radiologist implants in a relatively short procedure. This can be a complicated decision and also depends on the overall quality and expectancy of life. In some cases, when quality of life is poor, one can humanely say no to it all and opt for palliative or comfort care; there is no such thing as "must" when it comes to this juncture in life. Implanted artificial heart valves usually require lifelong blood thinning (aka anticoagulation). In these cases, the INR should be a bit higher, in the 2.5–3.5 range. Pig or cow valves do not usually require the same level of blood thinning as mechanical valves and an aspirin will often do.

The issue of preventing stokes in the elderly who may have had a transient ischemic attack (TIA) or prior stroke is complex and beyond the scope of this book. Please call AHCPR Publications for a readable, unbiased, government-commissioned summary about stroke prevention (800-358-9295 to order). You could also search the Internet. A plain old aspirin a day is usually the first-line therapy. Some have bought into the idea that a drug called Aggrenox (combination of lower-dose aspirin and dipyridamole) is marginally better, but just about all unbiased guidelines favor plain aspirin first. The new clot busters that you will read about such as TPA (Tissue Plasminogen Activators) are highly problematic in the elderly. First, the stroke must be caught within the first few hours and your loved one would have to be rushed to the nearest ER quickly. Any unstable medical picture or high blood pressure or history of bleeding would preclude its use. TPA also has not been studied well in the nursing home population. Only in an exceptional case would TPA be a consideration.

The so-called "statin" medications that lower the bad cholesterol have proved themselves in the elderly. Even my nihilistic medication tendencies take a backseat to preventing further cardiovascular damage with these medications. They include drugs like atorvastatin (Lipitor), simvastatin (Zocor), and pravastatin (Pravachol) to name a few. One should have a bona fide diagnosis of hyperlipidemia, usually but not always coupled with a prior event like a heart attack or stroke. Liver function tests need to be watched periodically, particularly at the beginning of treatment. Some of these drugs may be marginally better than others, but nowadays it's the insurance plan (Medicare Part D) that determines which will be reimbursed. Again, if someone has a poor life expectancy or is in the process of dying, there is no need to continue these medications. It sounds so obvious, but physicians are notorious for insisting that when people die, they die with a normal cholesterol!

Diuretic medications (aka water pills) are still the mainstay of treating congestive heart failure. These include plain vanilla furosemide (Lasix), bumetanide (Bumex), and torsemide (Demadex). Lasix is usually preferred for starters since it is cheap and usually well tolerated. Be sure the physician is monitoring kidney function and potassium levels after starting or increasing the dose. If the Lasix isn't doing the job, there are a few alternatives. One can switch to Bumex or Demadex. The absorption by the stomach of Lasix can be erratic, but these second-line expensive medications are absorbed more completely. The addition of a medication called metolazone (Zaroxolyn) can effect a quick loss of fluid, but be careful—severe potassium deficiency and/or dehydration is not uncommon. If your parent is being treated with metolazone, it is preferable that a kidney or heart specialist be involved. Also be sure that the drug is used sparingly, like a few times *a week* while the physician closely watches the kidney function and potassium levels via blood tests. Occasionally intravenous diuretics will do the trick when oral medications won't. Intravenous therapy can be achieved at the home if there is staff support, but commonly occurs in the hospital, too.

Most doctors also treat congestive heart failure with medications called ACE inhibitors or ARBs. This is especially true in diabetics for whom these drugs can also prevent kidney damage. The caveat here is that the drugs can paradoxically damage kidney function and raise potassium levels so they should be monitored as well. On occasion, ACE inhibitors also cause a nasty dry cough so if you notice that, please do ask if your parent is receiving an ACE inhibitor. If so, then consider a switch to an ARB that should provide the benefits but not the cough.

Antidepressants (and Appetite Stimulants)

While antidepressants might have been the most underused class of medications at one time, they now border on the most overused. Studies show that up to two-thirds of nursing home residents show symptoms of depression; however, not all of them need antidepressants. Many residents, especially those who are aware of the implications of being in a nursing home, will develop an adjustment disorder; they are having trouble getting used to the changes in their lives. Others may have suffered a recent loss and are going through the normal processes of bereavement and grieving. Still others have what we call dysthymia, which in my experience is a very common diagnosis in nursing homes. Dysthymia is a chronic sense of sadness or negativity that has likely been present for years. These are the folks that see the world as a glass half-empty rather than half-full. While some with these problems may go on in time to develop depression, there *is* a formal definition of major depression as outlined in the DSM-IV (*Diagnostic and Statistical Manual of Mental Disorders*).

People who suffer from major depression experience pervasive sadness or loss of interest for at least two weeks. In addition—and this is what really separates those with milder forms of depression from major depression—they have what we call neuro-vegetative signs. Their emotional distress begins to spill over and harm their health. The next chapter discusses depression in more detail with examples of some of these symptoms. Suffice it to say that while a true mood disorder (like major depression) often warrants treatment with medications, many other syndromes do not. Dementia with symptoms of depression is a particularly tough nut to crack; the resident often does not express herself clearly to identify the feelings of sadness per se. It is also this group that may be more prone to side effects.

Two main issues with the antidepressants besides expense and whether they are even needed are how long they take to work and the side effects one can develop from them. Even in young people, these medications can take two to three weeks and in the elderly the clinical saw is to give them between four to six weeks. This is a long period of time, especially if someone is losing weight or otherwise fading away. The major side effects of this group of medications are that they can paradoxically cause confusion, dizziness, weakness, and lethargy. Most of them can also cause low-level stomach symptoms such as nausea, flatulence, or diarrhea. These effects are not true of all people or of all antidepressants, but are at least a consideration if changes occur soon after starting.

A clinical maxim in geriatrics is "start low and go slow." Doses are usually about half the starting dose for younger people. Don't forget that while all the antidepressants on the market have been

FDA approved as being more effective than placebos (sugar pills), they are not more effective by much. We as geriatricians often care for nursing home residents in whom the diagnosis of major depression is not a slam dunk, and we consider the pros and cons of treating empirically—i.e., starting the medication and looking for an effect. I will prescribe them for a limited period of time and ask the family to give me feedback in a month's time to see if there has been any improvement. Of course, in parallel I am also observing and asking the staff to observe. The wonderful thing about nursing homes is that I am sharing the residents' environment with them. If I see them buying extra snacks at the canteen, I know they are eating better. If I see them at the weekly sing-alongs, I know they are socializing again.

One wonders if someone has been on an antidepressant for years how much good it is doing them. This underscores the federal government's new demands that we try to wean these and other psychoactive medications at least twice within a year. There better be a good reason *not* to attempt to wean though the full recourse the surveyors have is not yet clear. What irks me is when I find a resident with very advanced Alzheimer's disease who cannot speak or otherwise interact but is still on an antidepressant that has been carried along just because no one thought of stopping it. The person may be so debilitated that there is no way to gauge a positive effect of the medication. For all these reasons, less in the way of medications can really be more.

If your loved one is taking an antidepressant, let's run through the families of these drugs. The oldest two groups are almost obsolete. The first is the MAO inhibitors, named for the types of brain chemistry enzymes they can inhibit. Due to detrimental interactions with certain kinds of foods, these medications entail dietary restrictions. Psychiatrists use them only for severely resistant cases and rarely at that. The other group is known as the tricyclics. Amitriptyline (Elavil) still shows up in younger patients' medicine cabinets but in the elderly causes sedation, dry eyes, glaucoma, constipation, and incontinence.

Needless to say, the tricyclics rarely appear anymore on drug lists in nursing homes. Occasionally, doctors prescribe modified tricyclics called desipramine and nortriptyline. They are cheap and certainly less problematic than others in this group. They also have the possible side benefits of treating the neuropathy of diabetes and can decrease the frequency of urination a tad in those with overactive bladders.

The most commonly prescribed antidepressants are the so-called SSRIs (abbreviation for selective serotonin reuptake inhibitors). These are still in their heyday and Prozac was the first on the block in 1988. Since then there have been several more released (Paxil, Zoloft, Celexa, Lexapro, to name a few) and each is making its maker the richer for it. Drug detail people and my colleagues who have succumbed to the temptations of the pharmaceutical industry will try to tell you one is better than the next, but don't listen. They each can be about 15–20% more effective than a placebo and cause similar side effects of confusion, electrolyte disorders (mostly a low sodium level), loss of libido, and can exacerbate mania if the patient happens to have bipolar disorder (formerly known as manic-depressive disorder). By and large, they are pretty safe. The main question remains, are they doing any good? And even if they are beneficial, must they be kept going forever? Depression tends to be a cyclical disease and younger patients receive about six to nine months of treatment before weaning off. Obviously it depends on the severity and history of the depression. The recommendation for the elderly is to prescribe for about nine to twelve months and then attempt to wean. A significant recurrence of depression after this usually buys a longer or permanent regimen of an antidepressant. The other antidepressants comprise an assortment. You should be familiar with a few of the unusual properties of some of these.

For example, buproprion (Wellbutrin) can, in rare cases, cause seizures and hypertension, but if your parent has either of these conditions at baseline, it would not be a good choice. Venlafaxine (Effexor) can cause high blood pressure, though not commonly. Duloxetine (Cymbalta) is fairly new and seems to have an effect on diabetic nerve pain (neuropathy) and is FDA approved for that as well as depression. While more and more psychiatrists are diagnosing ADD at later ages, the use of methylphenidate (Ritalin) in nursing homes is unrelated. Geriatricians and others in the know have prescribed this medication for years for depression when the clock is running, so to speak. As an antidepressant it has some salutary effects. The difference is that it is said to work quickly rather than the month or more the standard antidepressants take. Cardiologists warned about cardiac side effects and high blood pressure but the medication is safer than first thought. I wouldn't give it to someone just getting over a heart attack or who has a heart rhythm irregularity or who has high blood pressure that is very difficult to control. The classic case for Ritalin would be an older person who has just fractured her hip, sails through surgery, but just when the therapy should begin in earnest, starts feeling very down and just won't play ball. The clock can run out pretty quickly on her; the nursing home justifies Medicare payment for the stay only if the resident does a certain number of minutes of therapy a day. So two or three days of "not feeling like" therapy can spell disaster. I have prescribed Ritalin in this situation. For sure, one needs also to enlist a multidimensional approach that involves the physical therapist, family, social worker, and perhaps a psychologist. Does Ritalin work? I'd have to say it's a case-by-case story, what we sometimes call "empirical." In other words, the data supports its use, but the percentages are not very high and many will not respond. So ask the physician to consider a trial if the potential benefits outweigh the risks.

Mirtazapine (Remeron) is one of the few antidepressants that can by itself cause weight gain. Since weight loss is very common in the elderly who are depressed, this can be a plus. Dieticians and nursing home administrators love it; unexpected weight loss is a black mark against a home when it comes to survey time. Just be careful on a few scores. First, the weight gain can be associated with fluid retention and swelling of the limbs (edema). Second, it is a fairly sedating medication so it is best given at night. Third, I have seen it requested by some dieticians simply as an appetite stimulant. If you had to use a pure appetite stimulant, mirtazapine would not be top choice.

The most common choice for a pure appetite stimulant is megestrol (Megace). Megestrol is a female sex hormone that has been approved by the FDA for weight loss only for AIDS and cancer patients. While is does cause mild weight gain in elderly nursing home residents, research has never shown it to extend lives or the quality of lives. In fact, very little research regarding appetite stimulants in this population has been done. Nursing homes tend to push them because they can be "dinged" by surveyors for weight loss. I have read the latest federal guidelines on weight loss and they are thankfully dubious on the benefits of appetite stimulants. Megestrol can cause blood clots in the legs and diabetes so there is literally no free lunch. Dronabinol (Marinol) is another appetite stimulant on the market and is derived from marijuana. It is, like megestrol, only approved in AIDS patients. I do confess to using these medications on *rare* occasions but only after I discuss the larger picture of decline with family and informing them of all risks if they still wish to proceed with a medication trial. For more on weight loss and its evaluation, see chapter 7.

Medications for Dementia

The first antidementia drug was developed in the mid-1980s and the last ten years have witnessed several more that have proved to be safer. These are drugs that are supposed to reharness the horsepower of the damaged brain. They are officially approved only for Alzheimer's disease, though you will see psychiatrists and neurologists among others apply them to people with other forms of dementia. The studies are fairly convincing that these medications improve some of the damaged domains of the brain such as memory, orientation, and ability to execute a task. The disappointment has been that the improvement occurs more on tests than in real life.

The goal of any treatment in the frail nursing home patient is to improve *function*. Does the improvement on a mental function test (a poor man's IQ test) translate into the person being able to do more for him- or herself? While I hate to be a party pooper, I can only offer that it's a case-by-case affair once again. I'm underwhelmed time and again by these expensive drugs and I just don't think there's any data that compels me to use them in frail nursing home residents. I do work together with families and explain to them why I feel that way and why we stopped them for my own father.

My father is seventy-nine years old and has had Alzheimer's for about eight or nine years. While the specific Alzheimer's drugs did very little for him, small doses of antidepressants and antipsychotics have worked wonders along the way. My dad's case has reinforced to me that each person's journey into old age, and especially into dementia, is unique. There are no absolutes and no magic bullets but keep an open mind.

The major group of Alzheimer's medications is the acetylcholinesterase inhibitors. That's a fancy way to say that the drugs slow down the natural breakdown of a certain brain chemical called acetylcholine. Loss of acetylcholine, most researchers now say, is not the *cause* of Alzheimer's but may be relevant in some of the symptoms, such as memory loss. The major side effect of these drugs is a loss of appetite that can cause significant weight loss.

The exemplars of this class are donepezil (Aricept), rivastigmine (Exelon), and galantamine (Razadyne). If you and your parent's doctor decide to stick with one of these or try them anew, aim for the lowest dose since a higher dose increases the risk of weight loss and other side effects. The drug companies are also putting out lots of data that the medications can modify some of the more disturbing behavioral symptoms of dementia such as agitation (despite recent *New England Journal of Medicine* articles and editorials to the contrary). Remember the same caveat that just because some measures on some tests improve, the utility of these medications to lessen these awful symptoms is less than great. The FDA has *never* approved use of these drugs for the behavioral challenges of Alzheimer's and has never approved their use in non-Alzheimer's dementia.

The most recent addition to the antidementia club is a medication that works on another brain chemical receptor and is known as an NMDA-receptor antagonist. Now forget that piece of trivia but recall that the FDA approved memantine (Namenda) only for moderate to severe Alzheimer's. It can be used in combination with the other family of antidementia drugs (the pro-acetylcholine medications). My strong advice is if you *are* going to allow the physicians to use an anti-Alzheimer's drug, please don't have them start *both* at the same time. *This is a general principle for many classes of drugs.* Avoid starting multiple drugs at the same time. First, if benefits accrue, you won't know which is responsible. Second, and more likely, if side effects such as confusion or a rash ensue, the medical team won't know which to stop.

If the FDA has not approved any of these medications for behavioral (as opposed to cognitive) symptoms of dementia, then what has it approved? The unfortunate answer is *none*! Part has to do with how difficult it is to do good research in a nursing home population and part has to do with lack of efficacy of anything available. Now just as a reminder, it is not illegal for a physician to prescribe a medication for a non-FDA-approved condition. Aricept can be prescribed for a non-Alzheimer's dementia such as that caused by multiple strokes. But the physician may be standing on thin ice to do so and should there be a bad outcome, the first question would be, Was the doctor meeting the standard of sound medical practice? Talk about cognitive dissonance!

The problem with agitation caused by dementia is that it is not only common, but can be severe and distressing to staff, family, and the resident. Since no medication is approved, there may be some leeway in a compassionate use sense. In other words, the cure may be worse than the disease but if the agitation is severe, one will try even chicken soup and the FDA be damned. The most compelling data favors judicious doses of antipsychotic medications. The favorable studies were not landmark cases by any stretch of the imagination, but they do suggest some utility. As a class of medications, the antipsychotics have received bad press over the years so it really comes down to a risk/benefit discussion. I look at their use as being similar to using narcotics such as morphine in people with pain or who are dying. Enough morphine can slow respirations and perhaps hasten death, but we never use it to achieve those ends. We use it because the goal is to alleviate pain and suffering. By the same token, many of those with advanced dementia suffer from severe agitation that can physically injure them and the staff. The behaviors also upset and injure the family emotionally. The use of high enough doses of any sedating medication can cause pneumonia and/or death. As long as everyone understands that this is a possible outcome, most physicians who take the time can talk the family into accepting those risks. The goal, once again, is not stupor or death but comfort and palliation.

The most common medications in this class are haloperidol (Haldol), risperidone (Ripserdal), olanzapine (Zyprexa), quetiapine (Seroquel), aripiprazole(Abilify), and ziprasidone (Geodon). While results were not conclusive, some studies have shown an increased rate of death and/or strokes in patients with dementia who take these medications. *The Physicians' Desk Reference* (PDR) labels these medications with a black box warning for exactly this reason. The other major side effect of these medications is worsening of diabetes or causing it in someone with a predisposition. In our home, we temporarily monitor blood sugars in any resident who newly receives an antipsychotic. Another problem with this class are so-called movement disorders (tremors, stiffness, shuffling gait) or "extrapyramidal" side effects. These were more common with the older medications like haloperidol, but can occur with the newer ones just mentioned.

The most dreaded of all side effects is tardive dyskinesia. T.D., as it's known, is vexing because once developed it *can* be irreversible. T.D. is the involuntary movement of certain parts of the body. Lip smacking and rocking of the trunk are just some examples. Most often, T.D. occurs after many years of relatively high doses of antipsychotics. It is more common in psychiatric patients, such as schizophrenics, who reside in state hospitals and are treated with high doses over many years. Some years ago, I cared for a woman from the former Soviet Union who had been a political prisoner. According to her family, she was regularly injected with "tranquilizers" while in prison. In retrospect, we determined these "tranquilizers" must have been antipsychotics. When she came to our home, she had the worst T.D. that I had ever seen. Her face not only contorted in rhythmic twisting, her whole body rocked back and forth and she could barely eat. The injections had stopped years before, but the effect was permanent. A friend of mine who is a lawyer and nobly represents residents of nursing homes and state hospitals tells me that Massachusetts requires informed consent before allowing a physician to use such medications. While this rule is widely ignored (possibly out of ignorance), it can be enforced when someone is lucky enough to have an advocate.

So what is a person to do? Allow your family member to receive these medications or not? You probably guessed the answer: case-by-case discussion. At least now you know the background and can ask the right questions. You should also know that different homes have different practices. In our home, we have two nursing units reserved for residents with moderate to advanced dementia. On these units, some of the agitated behaviors are expected and other residents are not cognizant enough to be upset by them. We use fewer medications even if it means more residents with aggressive behaviors.

If the nursing home tells you that transfer to another unit is warranted, due diligence is important, but don't fight too hard. Usually it's for the best and that's not just the party line talking. The units with more demented residents may not be the most attractive to you and may actually scare you, but they have better staffing and the staff is more patient…at least in my experience.

Do I personally prescribe antipsychotics? Of course I do, but

I do so cautiously and only after talking to staff and family. I do follow the rules of trying to wean the medications at least twice a year unless there's a very compelling reason not to.

Are there other medications besides the antipsychotics? Yes, and the psychiatrists that consult at the home will use some of them. This raises the thorny issue about proper use of consultants, which I will address in chapter 7. For now, know that there about five or ten other medications or classes of medications to treat agitated behaviors in dementia. Again, none has been FDA approved for this purpose. Benzodiazepines are a class of antianxiety medications. The older ones such as diazepam (Valium) should probably not be used. They last too long in the body and can accumulate quickly in the bloodstream. Newer ones such as lorazepam (Ativan) and alprazolam (Xanax) are shorter acting and can be worth a try to relieve some symptoms. If they don't work, I would quickly remove them and try something else. Some geriatric psychiatrists prescribe one of the antiseizure medications like carbamazepine (Tegretol), divalproex (Depakote), or gabapentin (Neurontin). I am spectacularly unimpressed with their use and the studies have been disappointing. These would be my last choice and only if desperate. One must monitor Depakote closely for liver inflammation and Tegretol for low blood counts by drawing blood tests. Many physicians forget this or never learned it, and if your parent is taking one of these, you should ask about the monitoring. It is also your right to question a certain treatment. If you get in a tussle with the physician, ask him or her to provide documentation that the proposed drug works and see what they say. It might even necessitate calling in the medical director for another opinion or switching to him or her as the physician of record.

Some of the agitation manifests itself in hypersexuality. I have seen both males and females exhibiting these behaviors, including masturbating in public, fondling other residents and/or staff, and exposing themselves. There is a fine line between the normal need for sexual release that is human nature and behaviors that cross the line. Perhaps simply escorting a resident to his or her room is enough, and behind closed doors they can fulfill their sexual urges. In my experience, staff is notoriously uncomfortable with this whole issue. Many of our staff are from socially conservative cultures and the idea of even talking about sex is alien. I do sit down with the staff and try to transcend the morality issue; I prefer to gun for the practical approach. I always have a senior female staff person with me, such as the director of nursing, to underscore how important a problem we are facing. The take-home message to staff is that we should utilize a uniform behavioral approach.

Certainly some of the sexuality is directed at others who may not consent. Everyone who encounters the resident is instructed to take him or her aside discreetly and let him or her know that they are being "watched." We usually use a hand signal like pointing to the eyes to indicate we are watching. When this is done frequently enough, it usually works. We also reward "good" behavior and praise the resident if they have gone part of the day without resorting to the disturbing behavior.

If the approach fails and medications are needed, I usually opt for an SSRI antidepressant first. As mentioned, one of the side effects is loss of libido and this can be used to our advantage. I always notify the family, especially since it may involve another resident. There are legal issues of consent as well. The other trick is to try an estrogen patch or estrogen medication for the male resident. The female sex hormone somehow decreases libido in men. There are some individual case reports and retrospective data that this helps. I personally am not a big believer, but I have resorted to it on occasions when all else fails. If nothing works, my job is to protect the other residents and staff. Transfer out of the nursing home may be necessary. Alas, this is where it gets interesting as there are few psychiatric units (and due to budget cuts, fewer as we speak) that accept such residents. State hospitals with geriatric units are an unappetizing possibility. Fortunately, these are rare occurrences.

Diabetic Medications

If there's one field that has seen an explosion of medications, it's diabetes. Treating diabetes used to be an effortless affair. There was *one* family of oral medications that simply was referred to as "oral agents" and everyone knew that meant sulfonylureas, such as chlorpropamide (Diabinese). Diabinese is barely used now but a profusion of "me, too" drugs has taken its place. The newer ones are safer, and glipizide (Glucotrol) and glyburide (Micronase or Diabeta) are examples of this class. There are several other families of oral medications and each work differently. A discussion here could not do the topic justice, but please search the web or visit the AGS Foundation for Health in Aging at www .healthinaging.org/public_education/diabetes/medications.php for an excellent summary. This site also summarizes the plethora of insulins that are now available.

For now, a few general principles will suffice. First, if you had to choose between a blood sugar (blood glucose) that is a bit high and a blood sugar that is too low, always take the former. Monitoring diabetes has become easier with the advent of finger-stick glucose-monitoring machines. This palm-sized instrument is used by all nursing homes and hospitals and most diabetics use them at home, too. Researchers on type I young onset diabetes have shown conclusively that "tight" control (i.e., running blood sugars as low as it is safe to do) prevents long-term complications such as kidney, heart, and eye disease. These studies, however, were not performed on nursing home residents who mostly suffer from type II maturity onset diabetes. Moreover, are we really seeking to prevent long-term complications when the average survival in a nursing home is less than a year? By the same token, are we looking to maximize longevity as much as the quality of your loved one's life? Tight control means more episodes of low blood sugar (hypoglycemia) and these can be dangerous in the frail elderly who cannot respond to the usual cues of an impending hypoglycemic reaction. What compounds the problem is that the very well-meaning endocrinologist (or primary-care provider) who saw your parent in the hospital was aiming for "tight" control. Sugars *that* low are just not practical or safe in long-term care. Tight control often means four finger sticks every day. I don't think many of us would relish being stuck in the fingers with a sharp needle that often. Often the hospital orders for insulin and other diabetic medications are simply carried over reflexively at the nursing home. It might be worth your asking *and* suggesting that the doctor reverts to the program in place before the hospital.

The second principle is to keep it simple. While many younger people living at home take three or four medications for diabetes daily plus insulin, this complex a regimen may not be necessary in the nursing home. Some can be managed on an old warhorse sulfonylurea like glipizide. If your parent is on an insulin regimen, can the oral agents that failed to control the diabetes simply be stopped? Again, we're not looking to prolong life or squeeze out ever-lower numbers (or at least we shouldn't be). When I was a resident at a fancy teaching hospital in Boston, it used to be said of the residents in training that perhaps we knew how to let a terminal patient succumb, but he had to die with a normal glucose and potassium! A simpler regimen of one or two injections daily may suffice. Your parent will be eternally grateful if you can avoid superfluous insulin injections and finger sticks each day. For those on hospice care or for whom death is expected, we either stop the finger sticks or greatly reduce the frequency. In many of my stable residents, hospice or not, I reduce the finger sticks to once or twice a week.

Stomach Medications and Antiacids

As an acid reflux sufferer, I share others' relief when the flames of heartburn are doused. I can also tell you that the newer antiacid medications are among the most overused on the market. The problem is that since these medications have relatively few side effects, doctors often prescribe them prophylactically with very little data or evidence to support this practice. Doctors that treat in hospitals are particularly guilty. Costs increase and there is a theoretical problem in lowering the acid content of the stomach too much. Absence of normal acid can affect the absorption of other medications or certain vitamins *and* be a risk for pneumonia. In a recent study presented at a nursing home medical directors' meeting, a researcher scanned the charts of ninety-eight residents and found that almost two-thirds were on a proton pump inhibitor such as omeprazole (Prilosec), Protonix, Prevacid, or Nexium. Of that number, only half had a diagnosis that justified the medication. A consultant pharmacist worth his or her salt (recall that their reviews are mandated by law) will pick up on this and query the use of the medication. Some doctors will stop the meds and others will ignore the suggestion. One hopes that with the tightening of the new federal regulations against unnecessary medications, more doctors will see the light and just say no.

Pulmonary Medications and Treatments

Bronchodilators represent the most common issue relating to treatment of lung disease. Different bronchodilators work in slightly different ways, but all "dilate" or enlarge the airways to allow more oxygen to get into the lungs and be delivered to the body. Classically, these are used for pure asthma. Asthmatics are usually on the younger side and go through pulmonary function tests (PFTs) that determine whether bronchodilators improve their airways. Most asthmatics do improve and use a handheld device called an inhaler with medications like albuterol (Proventil), and/or ipratropium (Atrovent). Sometimes physicians prescribe these combined with inhaled anti-inflammatory medications called steroids (for example, Advair Diskus). Inhalers take some coordination and skill to use. For best use, you also need to hold your breath after inhaling. I vividly recall a woman for whom I cared who was in her midforties and had severe asthma. No matter what inhaler I threw at her, she kept on wheezing. Finally one day I asked her to bring her inhaler to the office and asked her to demonstrate its use. She promptly held it up and "spritzed" herself around her neck and arms as if it were perfume. Not a molecule went into her lungs!

While frail elderly can be *instructed* in the proper technique, my experience is that very few inhale the medications properly. A device called a "spacer" can be helpful. This is a four- or five-inch tube that hooks up to the opening of the inhaler and allows the user to inhale from a chamber so she need not coordinate the squeezing of the inhaler with taking a breath and holding it. Children use them to good effect. For some reason, many nursing homes don't utilize spacers and, to make matters worse, Medicare Part D does not appear to pay for them. It might be worth you buying it yourself (about twenty dollars and can be bought at most drugstores or online) or asking the pharmacy at the nursing home to purchase it and charge for it.

Even with spacers, most inhalers don't work well, particularly if your parent has any cognitive impairment (read dementia). The staff then resorts to nebulizer treatments. These are essentially the same medications but in liquid form that are aerosolized and propelled into the lungs by a nebulizer machine—through a mask or "peace pipe" apparatus. It tends to deliver more drug into the lungs but is expensive, noisy, and more time-consuming since each treatment takes fifteen minutes of nursing time. Luckily, one can tell clinically (that is, by observing the person and listening to their lungs with a stethoscope) if the inhaler or the nebulizer is working. The wheezing and shortness of breath should diminish.

The looming question, though, is if asthma is not as common in the elderly, why do we use so many bronchodilators? I should add a caveat that while pure asthma is *not* common, chronic obstructive pulmonary disease (COPD) can have elements of asthma and/or emphysema mixed in. A patient with COPD then probably deserves a trial of a bronchodilator, but like all medications, if it's not helping, ask the doctors to stop it. The other kicker is that doctors in the hospital and nursing home will prescribe a bronchodilator for anyone who breathes a little funny or has a cough or congestion. This results in overuse and overkill. If the medication is doing any good, you'll know very soon when it is stopped. It can always be restarted in a hurry. Asthma itself is often cyclical or intermittent and just because it helps one week does not mean it will be needed forever.

Oral steroids like prednisone have also become a mainstay in treating younger people with pure asthma. Steroids have multiple short- and long-term complications and should be used sparingly. They usually don't work in older people with shortness of breath. When they *do* work, they can be life-saving. The two most dreaded short-term complications are elevation of blood sugars, especially in diabetics, and the development of acute confusion—so-called steroid psychosis. If you know your parent has responded to steroid medication positively (and they can be used for many different illnesses) in the past, please let the physician know this.

Kidney Medications

This group of medications doesn't really work on the kidneys but helps modify other systems in the body that go awry in kidney disease. Because there are two kidneys, there is lots of room for error; both kidneys need to be severely damaged for these other systems to go bad. To get a quick gauge of how bad things are you might want to ask about a few lab numbers. The creatinine and less important the blood urea nitrogen (BUN) are measures of kidney function. Any creatinine over 1.5 or 2 signifies a significant problem, but I have plenty of patients with a creatinine of 2 or 2.5 who remain stable for years and have no discernible problems. The tendency, however, is for there to be progressive deterioration once the number reaches the mid 2s or 3. Because this number is highly variable depending on the size and age of the patient, a better measure is called the creatinine clearance or glomerular filtration rate (GFR). The normal level is over one hundred and kidney disease usually starts as it begins to fall below sixty. One best measures GFR by collecting urine for twenty-four hours and sending it to a lab. This, it turns out, is highly impractical and often requires a catheter inserted in the bladder that no one likes. A more convenient way is to calculate the GFR based on weight, age, and the creatinine number. Most labs will do that and send it along with the blood work. Just remember that while this is handy, it's just not that accurate.

If one has established significant kidney disease, beware that it can affect two major systems. The first is the balance between calcium, phosphate, and the bones of the body. If kidney disease throws this balance off, the result can be a glandular problem known as hyperparathyroidism and eventually a dangerously high calcium level. The treatment for this involves numerous expensive possibilities such as Rocaltrol, Sensipar, Renagel, Zemplar, Fosrenol, PhosLo, Hectorol, etc. The much cheaper Tums (yes, *that* Tums) can sometimes be used, too. In general, a kidney specialist should help manage this. Though in some rural areas, access may be limited and a primary-care doctor can do the honors.

The second system that kidney disease affects is the blood-forming unit in the bone marrow. The kidney contains a hormone called erythopoietin that helps the bone marrow do its job. When the kidney begins to fail (we're talking about a creatinine usually approaching three or more and a GFR of less than twenty or thirty), there are three types of injections one can give that take the place of erythopoietin. It is only suggested to use the injections (Epogen, Procrit, or Aranesp) if anemia is present to the extent that it causes weakness and lack of oxygen delivery. If only it were that simple. First, now that Medicare Part D is paying for the drug, the physician must go through some paperwork to prove that it's really needed and there is enough iron in the body for the hormone to utilize. The paperwork is not too demanding and actually is good at weaning out who needs and who doesn't need. Second, because of new safety concerns it's not clear who needs the hormones anyway. *The New York Times* and other papers recently ran front-page articles based on new research. The conclusions of the research were that the gospel of these hormones being beneficial to patients with kidney failure was not infallible after all.

In certain circumstances, the patients who received the hormones actually faired worse. Patients who received the hormones for other reasons, namely that they had anemia due to cancer, actually declined and their tumors grew faster! *The Times* also found that some physicians accept financial incentives to prescribe the medications, which is not good news for this multibillion-dollar industry. The take-home message is clear. The FDA and Medicare will be restricting these hormones more and more and that's probably a good thing. You may not need to intervene. There are some patients the hormones help, but be inquisitive if you see one of these hormone injections listed on your parent's regimen.

Pain Medications

Pain is omnipresent in long-term care. Low estimates are that 50% of residents have chronic pain; higher estimates range up to 80%. About 15% have persistent pain (always in pain). While we physicians wish to diagnose the cause of pain, we too often neglect treating the pain itself. This is one area in which the state and federal surveyors have lightened up and encourage aggressive pain management before a firm diagnosis can be pinned down. Sometimes we never elucidate the cause of the pain, but we nevertheless treat it. The nursing profession is decidedly ahead of the medical profession. Almost all acute and non-acute settings see pain as a vital sign, like temperature and blood pressure. Nurses must perform pain-rating scales that are easy, quantitative, and informative. The bugaboo with aggressive treatment was and in some corners remains the fear of frail elders becoming addicted to narcotic pain medications. Before we explore the types of pain medications available, let's dispense with this old canard.

Most experts agree that addiction is the compulsive use of a medication for purposes other than for what it was intended. For example, rather than a narcotic controlling pain, the addict seeks it out for its high. The addict often uses dishonest and devious means of obtaining more drugs. His or her behaviors become socially suspect and maladaptive. When a doctor prescribes morphine, for example, to treat a chronic arthritic knee that has failed any other mode of treatment, in anyone's book that is a legitimate medical use of the drug. As long as the doctor continues to prescribe it, monitor it, and is convinced that the medication is improving function, then it *cannot* represent addiction. It is typical that as one takes a narcotic for medical reasons, the doctor may need to increase the dose. The body's natural receptors to narcotic medications sometimes become tolerant and higher doses are needed to achieve the same effect. This does *not* equal addiction.

While there are certainly other medications to try before reaching for a narcotic, many of them are fraught with side effects. Do not view narcotics as last-ditch medications only for those writhing in pain. If the doctor balances the risks and benefits, narcotics will often win out. Don't forget that there *are* nonpharmacological modalities of pain treatment. (We explored several of these in the discussion of PTs and OTs in chapter 5.) Physical and occupational therapists often guide those approaches.

The World Health Organization (WHO) took the lead several years ago on issues relating to pain. They summarized what others had been saying. Effective pharmacological pain control depends on the *right pill* at the *right dose* at the *right time*. The pill must be up to the job and adequate to the level of pain. It must be sufficient in quantity to do the job. It must be given on an around-the-clock basis. This latter point is crucial in nursing homes. Too often physicians write an order on a "prn" or "as needed" basis; the pill is given only if the patient complains of pain. So many residents of long-term care are confused and cannot voice their wishes that the prn pills are simply not given. If one always depends on the nurse to judge the severity of a resident's pain, we leave too much to chance. A standing routine dose is far preferred. Around those doses, it is appropriate to write a prn order for what we call breakthrough pain. For example, if one uses codeine to treat the pain from a wrist fracture, a proper order would be "thirty milligrams every six hours around the clock and thirty milligrams every four hours as needed for breakthrough pain."

As part of their campaign, the WHO published the "Three Step Analgesia Ladder." This tells us what the right drug is for the level of pain. The first step of the ladder is mild pain, for which acetaminophen (Tylenol) or a nonsteroidal anti-inflammatory is appropriate. Acetaminophen is limited by its toxicity to the liver; four grams per day (twelve tablets of regular strength or eight tablets of extra-strength) is the maximum dose. Do not underestimate the efficacy of acetaminophen. Placebo-controlled studies found it as good as ibuprofen (Motrin, Advil) for knee arthritis and it caused fewer side effects. Nonsteroidals have been much in the news due to the cardiac woes of Vioxx. There are plenty of others left on the market and most are over-the-counter. Nonsteroidals notoriously cause stomach ulcers and leg swelling and can at least temporarily worsen kidney function. I do use them on occasion in those with reasonable kidney function with an acute problem like a sprain or gout, but I will only write it for three days at most. Some studies support the use of an acid-blocker to protect the stomach for any prolonged nonsteroidal use.

The second rung of the WHO ladder is moderate pain. For this, we prescribe a nonnarcotic medication called tramadol (Ultram or Ultracet when combined with acetaminophen) that is about as potent as codeine. We also use combinations of acetaminophen with a narcotic: codeine (Tylenol #2, 3, or 4, depending on the dose of the codeine), hydrocodone (Vicodin), or oxycodone (Percocet or Roxicet). What you should notice is that even on step two of the ladder, we are into narcotic medications. You will also note the absence of acetaminophen combined with propoxyphene (Darvocet), and meperidine (Demerol). Due to side effects and lack of efficacy, these medications are considered much less desirable and many doctors refuse to prescribe them altogether. The second-rung drug doses are limited mostly by the maximum daily four-gram dose of the acetaminophen. Therefore, if these medications are not doing the trick and the patient is still in pain, we advance quickly to the third rung: severe pain.

This third level requires medications like morphine (usually as a generic short-acting MSIR and short-acting liquid Roxanol, or long-acting pills such as MS-Contin, Kadian, and Oramorph SR), oxycodone (short-acting OxyIR and short-acting liquid OxyFast, or as long-acting Oxycontin), hydromorphone (Dilaudid), and fentanyl (as generic or as the Duragesic patch). Not all physicians are comfortable prescribing these medications. If that is the case and the patient is also on hospice, the hospice doctors and nurses can be helpful and will see to it that treatment is appropriate. If not, then ask the medical director to intervene and/or ask for another physician. In this day and age, you cannot allow an uninformed or resistant physician to hold your loved one hostage to pain.

The preferred method for beginning rung-three treatment is

with short-acting oral medications like oxycodone (OxyIR or Oxy-Fast) or morphine (MSIR or Roxanol). When control of pain is achieved or close to being achieved, the physician should total the daily dose in milligrams needed and convert that into the longer-acting forms. For example, over the first three days of increasing doses to control pain, fifteen milligrams of oxycodone is used every six hours, that totals to sixty milligrams per day and we prescribe Oxycontin (long-acting), thirty milligrams every twelve hours, which totals sixty milligrams, too. It is proper to prescribe a breakthrough dose as needed (as opposed to the *only* order being as needed). Presumably, the nurses will have been trained to recognize nonverbal signs if the patient cannot voice her own complaints of pain. If you are in the room, and your loved one *is* in pain, by all means ask the nearest nurse for the breakthrough dose. Morphine can be prescribed in the same fashion.

The liquid preparations are absorbed similarly to the oral tablet but are useful in a few instances. They can be given easily if the patient has a PEG (percutaneous endoscopic gastrostomy) tube for feeding. If the resident does not swallow well, both Roxanol and OxyFast are in a highly concentrated liquid and can be absorbed from the mouth without having to swallow. They are very commonly used in hospice care. The formulations of narcotics are so varied and refined that injections are practically not needed. They are painful and only should be used for emergencies or if the oral medication is not available. This breaks with hospital tradition, but properly so.

The fentanyl (Duragesic) patch deserves special mention. While appealing in theory, the patch has very different rates of absorption in different people and is highly unpredictable. It is also very expensive. The patch is applied only every three days (every two days at the most) and takes about three or four of those intervals to reach the proper blood level of painkiller. For getting rid of pain quickly, it is highly problematic and I would not use it. If someone has been on a steady long-acting regimen for some time and wishes the convenience of an every three-day patch as opposed to pills, then one could convert. There are tables that will help the physician give the appropriate strength patch. Dolophine (methadone) has enjoyed a resurgence of late as an effective long-acting cheap narcotic. The dosing of it is far more complex than any other narcotic and few physicians besides pain specialists or those with a lot of experience should be prescribing it. One glance at the *PDR* will give you serious pause.

All narcotics cause some degree of constipation and a bowel softener and/or laxative needs to be prescribed to avoid problems down the road. I have patients who refuse narcotics altogether because of the fear of constipation! Narcotics often cause sedation and sleepiness. They can also cause confusion. This usually goes away after the first few days, but the dose can be lowered or the time interval between which it is given can be lengthened. If these side effects are so severe the patient cannot stay awake and cannot eat, an injected antidote known as naloxone (Narcan) can immediately reverse these side effects.

At each stage of the WHO ladder is listed the word "adjuvants." These are secondary medications that are sometimes used in tandem with the above medications to relieve pain, sometimes on their own. They are not typical analgesics. Some like gabapentin (Neurontin), carbamazepine (Tegretol), pregabalin (Lyrica), and divalproex (Depakote) are antiseizure medications. Others like amitriptyline (Elavil) and duloxetine (Cymbalta) are antidepressants. Mexilitene is a potent cardiac drug. These are almost all used for a condition called neuropathy, whether of the diabetic or the post-shingles variety. Neuropathic pain arises from nerves usually in the feet and legs, is vexing indeed, and often is not very responsive to narcotics. The literature in support of these medications is variable but a trial can be assayed as long as someone (i.e., the doctor) is really minding the store.

Another class of medications listed with the adjuvants is the steroid group of glucocorticoids exemplified by prednisone. Oncologists frequently use these to counter the pain of cancer after it has spread to bone. Their other major use is for a disease known as PMR (polymyalgia rheumatica). This is an unusual disease, but occurs primarily in older people and is marked by aching of the shoulders and hips. The pain can be so intense that patients cannot lift up their hands to comb their hair or to brush their teeth. Blood tests are abnormal and usually reflect an elevated erythrocyte sedimentation rate (ESR or sed rate) and anemia. Prednisone at the low dose of fifteen milligrams a day eases the pain within a day or two. PMR can be accompanied by a more serious condition called temporal arteritis that causes headaches and can affect vision. It is treated with much higher doses of prednisone and a rheumatologist is usually involved.

Especially for neuropathic pain, pain specialists sometimes need to be called in to offer an opinion and come up with other measures should medications fail. They may propose one or more epidural injections along the spine for pinched spinal nerves. They may propose a sympathectomy, a surgical procedure to interrupt the sympathetic nerve pathways, for other more complex nerve disorders. My advice here is to *tread carefully*. With all due respect, most pain doctors in my area are converted anesthesiologists and are in touch with their inner cowboy. They inject first and ask questions later. I cannot recall a frail nursing home patient who benefited in a sustained way from one of these procedures. For my money and for your money, you are better off with a physical medicine/rehabilitation doctor (physiatrist).

When it comes to pain, be aggressive as an advocate for your loved one. The state, the feds, good medical practice, good nursing practice, and the divinity itself will be on your side. Don't be afraid of narcotics. Your loved one will not become an addict. Remember the World Health Organization's ladder and if you "can't get no satisfaction," climb your own ladder up the administrative rungs of the home until you get satisfaction. I think you would want the same done for you. I know I would.

Other Medications and a Final Word from Your Sponsor

The other large group of medications is antibiotics. I will cover these in chapter 11 on infectious diseases in long-term care. The bottom line with all medications is that you should be looking for reasons to take people off of medications rather than slather more on. The average nursing home patient is on more than nine medications. This used to be the panic level but now has become quite a meaningless number. The more medications to hand out, the less time the nurses have to actually be nurses as opposed to pill-dispensing machines. Be aware that vitamins and alternative medications like Saint-John's-wort, ginko, etc., may sound great in theory, but if you request them, you'd better have darn good evidence that they work in a *significant* way. If you want the doctors to do their work, then please do *your* work and don't make *more* work for everyone.

If you feel, based on this book or other sources, that a medication is not needed or may be dangerous, call or meet with the doctor and ask him or her to stop it. More than likely, he or she will agree and a convergence of state surveyors and Medicare apparatchiks will already have speeded them in that direction (just FYI, the federal rule we're talking about here is called F-tag 329, and specifically refers to unnecessary medications). If you run up against a reluctant physician, you can appeal to the administrator and say that with the information you have now, you refuse to have the medication given to your loved one. That will most likely be honored and the medical director should be asked in to get the deed done. Alternatively, he or the actual attending physician may be able to explain to your satisfaction why the medication is indicated. Failing that and only in rare circumstances, you have a case for the ombudsman's office...not a card to play lightly, but one that you do hold in your hand.

7

Consultants and Specialists: More or Less?

One of the tenets of medicine is "first, do no harm." Or as Dr. Jerome Groopman (author and medical writer for *The New Yorker*) says, "Don't just do something...stand there!"

When do you absolutely need a specialist to see your parent? Can the nursing home recommend someone and is it worth the hassle and expense to send your loved one out in a rainstorm for a specialist's exam? Can you keep the same cardiologist your parent has seen for twenty years or should you use the one who goes to the nursing home? Is it necessary to have a wound specialist or a pain specialist when the home seems to be doing a good job? What about when something doesn't seem right? Should you complain to the medical director or take the matter into your own hands? Why would a psychiatrist be asked to see your mom when she only has a "mild case of Alzheimer's"? Can a hospice patient see a specialist? This chapter provides you with the ground rules to solve the age-old dilemma of when to get another opinion and when not to.

I'll come clean from the start: My bias is that in nursing homes, many consultants can be avoided. And why, you might ask, should they even be avoided? Isn't it worth having a second opinion? Aren't two heads better than one? In short, less is sometimes more. The general problem with nursing homes and second opinions is access and appropriateness. Most homes in the country do not have the luxury of an outside specialist coming into the home to do their exam. Residents must per force be sent by transportation to an office; it often involves great expense and potential discomfort to the resident. If the resident is not on Medicaid or a Medicare Part A stay, the expense to you may be hundreds of dollars in copays and transportation. If the resident is covered by one of those programs, the cost is to the government or the nursing home. If you can transport your family member yourself safely, then you may save money.

The expense to the home can also be considerable; many homes send an aide to accompany the resident. This is by no means universal, but we have learned the hard way at our home. Most doctor's offices are pristine places and don't appreciate a potentially boisterous person with Alzheimer's "sullying" their waiting room. I am only the messenger with this comment, so don't shoot me. A few specialists have even told me that they will see my residents only in an emergency room, which is a horrible and expensive solution.

An effective consultation depends on the amount of information that changes hands. The more the nursing home or attending physician provides, the more targeted and useful the evaluation is. I recently had a resident who simply couldn't live with the amount of arthritic knee pain she was having. I had tried everything I could medically and finally gave up and asked an orthopedist to see her for a possible steroid injection in the knee. I sometimes do these myself, but she has a severely arthritic knee and I wanted an expert. This particular orthopedist would only see her in the emergency room. While I usually call the consultant ahead of time, I had mixed up the day my patient was supposed to be seen and when I realized it, I paged the doctor right away. To his credit, he called me right back but said he had seen her already and shipped her back to the home. Though she is quite lucid and knew why she was there, she failed to emphasize the knee and began talking about every pain and ache she had had for the last year. I suppose the orthopedist became overwhelmed and only performed some X-rays that confirmed the arthritis.

So *no* injection and *no* value from the visit. One could argue that maybe her knee wasn't so bad after all or she would have focused on it. One could also argue that there was a breakdown in communication. Even with the best of intentions, the best notes, and copying the correct records to send, these kinds of things happen commonly. When we send someone sick to the emergency room for evaluation and admission to the hospital, call the ER ahead of time, *and* send all appropriate notes, the data is sometimes separated from the resident (including the all important living will!).

So what is the solution? Should we sacrifice all consultations due to these issues? Clearly not. Some doctor's offices are terrific, but the more that you can share with them ahead of time the better. If the nursing home physician takes the time to call or send records, all the better, but much like obtaining the list of discharge medications yourself, you might want to call the office ahead of time or go along in tow to advocate. The better scenario is that the consultant actually visits the home him or herself. My home is blessed in being relatively large so that the consultants will often have more than one person to see at a time, which makes the trip worth their while. Some of my consultants actually regard coming to the nursing home as a charitable good deed. I don't disabuse them of this notion if it gets them to stop by. I try to credential the specialists who actually *like* spending time with the elderly and can josh with them. They may not match your list of "top docs," but believe me, in the end they provide better service. Don't rely on someone who has taken care of your mom or dad for years. They may be out of touch with nursing home regulations and the basics of geriatric care. If the nursing home doctor is recommending someone else, consider going in that direction.

The advantages of such visits by the consultants at the home are numerous. First, they have ready access to the chart and all its trimmings *and* they have access to the staff who can usually fill them in on the resident. Second, it saves the resident from a sometimes cold, rainy, expensive, and bumpy ride to who knows where. It is not uncommon for those who go out to come back with nary a sheet of paper telling what transpired. Let us go through several types of specialists and try to plumb how useful they are and what their modus operandi is likely to be.

Podiatrists, Ophthalmologists, and Dentists

Most podiatrists come to the nursing home to do their work. They often appear at set times as determined by the allowed frequency of visits by the insurance company or Medicare. These visits are about every eight to nine weeks but if there is a compelling problem, the podiatrist may visit on an emergent basis. While many primary-care providers can take care of common foot and toe problems, open wounds on the foot or lower leg may warrant a podiatrist's opinion. Toe or foot ulcers (i.e., wounds) can turn bad in a hurry (especially in diabetics and people with poor circulation) and podiatrists are familiar with ways to take pressure off certain areas of the foot or toes and to order the correct type of shoes. Some podiatrists also specialize in wounds called "venous stasis ulcers" and can be asked in to render an opinion.

Ophthalmologists also often visit nursing homes. They sometimes bring their equipment with them or the home may have a small eye clinic room. Most homes have a policy of providing the new residents with routine eye care within a month of admission and then it is up to the eye doctor to determine follow-up. Getting an eye doctor to come in promptly for a new problem can be difficult. It means a special trip and their office practices are usually very busy. Most primary-care providers should be able to care for routine eye complaints like redness, dry eyes, and minor infections. More complex problems like double vision or sudden documented loss of vision in one eye warrant a specialist's visit and the home may need to send someone out. With actual visual loss, don't hesitate to be the squeaky wheel and push for an earlier appointment. Optometrists (not medical doctors per se but trained in diseases of the eye) in most states do routine eye exams, besides ordering the correct glasses, and it may be that at your parent's home, an optometrist in the home will be your best hope.

The dentist is an important member of the care team and not a few residents in long-term care have stopped eating and lost weight due to mouth pain. Many facilities have a dental suite and a dentist who comes in periodically or even several times a week. Others have mobile dentists whose specialty is geriatric dentistry. Like good podiatric service and eye care, dentistry is seen as essential to long-term care and facilities must ensure access. Our own suite has most of the equipment that a decent if slightly primitive office might have including an X-ray machine.

Psychiatrists and Psychologists

The next busiest consultant in long-term care is the psychiatrist. Dementia and depression are rampant in nursing homes. Most geriatricians feel skilled enough to care for the basic needs of residents beset by these problems. Most internists do not and often call in a psychiatrist. Why a psychiatrist for management of dementia and not a neurologist? That's just the way the cookie has crumbled over the years. While *diagnosis* of dementia may fall in the purview of the neurologist, the day-to-day *management* falls to the psychiatrist. It likely has to do with the fact that most of the medications used in these situations are psychiatric medications prescribed for schizophrenia and depression. Unfortunately, there rarely is "day-to-day" management. Many geriatric psychiatrists make long-term care only a part of their practice and tend to make their visits after hours. Because of this, they don't have contact with the daytime staff, who can be invaluable in clarifying the problem. It also makes it challenging to speak with the primary physician.

More often than not, the need for a consultation originates with the director of nursing, the social worker, or the administrator in "cover your behind" mode. If a resident has done anything dangerous to herself or others, has expressed any sexual interest in staff or residents, has voiced any intent to harm herself, or has wandered outside the building, the powers that be will strongly suggest or demand a psychiatric evaluation. Even if the primary physician doesn't think a psychiatric consultation is necessary, he or she will eventually be ground into submission. I can be pretty stubborn when it comes to trying to do things myself, but for the sake of the facility and minimizing our risk in what can be potentially (though rarely) disastrous circumstances, I mostly knuckle under to the worries of the "boss." But if I really think, for example, that a statement like "I'm so bored I could kill myself" is a turn of phrase and not a threat, then I need to examine the resident myself and write an extensive note saying why I think a psychiatrist's visit is not warranted.

There are several legitimate reasons to consult a psychiatrist. If the talk of suicide is perceived to be real (and sometimes it's awfully hard to tell), then it's a good thing to bring someone in soon. If that can't happen, a trip to an ER to see a psychiatric screener might be the ticket. The screener will decide if the person needs to be committed or, short of that, voluntarily signed into a psychiatric unit. Needless to say, hospitals have closed these units right and left and options are drying up. From the narrow viewpoint of the nursing home and liability, at least the home can say that they sniffed out a problem and did the right thing in referring the resident on for help. Resistant depression, which is to say depression that is not getting better with the usual antidepressants, generally earns a visit from a psychiatrist, too.

The most common reason for a consultation, and in some ways the least productive, is for the demented resident with agitation. As I discussed in chapter 6, the pharmacological approach here is hit-or-miss and there is precious little data to guide us. What exacerbates the difficulty is that good geriatric psychiatrists are hard to come by. By "good" I mean psychiatrists who do not feel the pressure to prescribe, who are willing to contact families, who sit down with the staff to understand what's at issue, and who are sensitive to the cultural nuances of the residents. At the risk of sounding politically incorrect, I have been at nursing homes made up of residents of a particular ethnic or racial group that utilized mostly nonnative, English-speaking psychiatrists. Some of the exchanges I have witnessed have left me bewildered. There appears to be little useful information being exchanged. This is, after all, a specialty that depends on verbal communication and tone. For sure, there are exceptions and my facility is blessed to have two very fine and patient psychiatrists, each of whom received their training overseas. The real world being what it is, keep aware that culture and language can factor into the usefulness of such a consultation.

My own consultant psychiatrists excluded, I have seen some pretty strange and potentially dangerous combinations of medications. It is not unusual to admit a resident from another facility who is on five psychoactive medications—two for dementia, two for agitation, and one for depression, at the least. How can one possibly know which is doing what and which side effect is from which drug? I have also seen a psychiatrist come into a home on a Saturday night, spend at most a few minutes with a resident, and then order a cocktail of drugs. The take-home point here is that a second opinion can be a lousy opinion; less is often more.

Some facilities have the benefit of a psychologist on staff. This is a nonphysician psychotherapist, who as opposed to using medications tries behavioral or talk therapy to help those in need. They can often be helpful and, like chicken soup, really can't hurt. The only problem I think I see is that the therapists tend to keep the therapy going ad infinitum and occasionally do so in demented residents who I don't think can really participate in ongoing therapy. This also raises billing and compliance issues at times. I personally find their work useful, especially in addressing staff reaction to certain behaviors, which is often half the battle.

Dermatologists, Surgeons, Orthopedists, Urologists, and ENTs

Dermatologists are in great demand and it is often difficult to attract them to a nursing home. Nevertheless, older people are rife with skin problems. Many competent physicians can address simple rashes, but if a rash is not responding to the usual ointments and creams, you might want to suggest a dermatologist's opinion. Psoriasis is one condition that can be resistant to treatment. There are newer, more aggressive ways to treat psoriasis in which dermatologists are expert. In later chapters, I address some skin conditions such as pressure ulcers and scabies (an infestation similar to lice), but the major reason to use a dermatologist in a nursing home is for the scourge of skin cancer. As to the dangers of solar exposure, the current population of elders was ignorant at best and sun-worshipping at worst. Tanning lotions eventually gave way to sunscreens, but not until the damage was done. On the other hand, sun exposure was good for vitamin D stores in the body and building stronger bones, so it wasn't a total loss. Some of my residents develop lesion after lesion and all are suspicious for skin cancers.

We used to take a more casual approach. We thought that our residents would *not* outlive their skin cancers; experience has taught us otherwise. Unless someone is truly in the last six months of life, it is worth jumping on suspected skin cancers early. Some of the more aggressive-looking lesions paradoxically turn out to be benign "seborrheic keratoses"; these do not need to be biopsied or removed unless they are a major cosmetic issue. Others are either squamous cell cancers or basal cell cancers (carcinomas). Often the biopsy is curative as the dermatologist succeeds in removing the entire lesion at the time of biopsy. Other times, he or she will need to come back with some equipment that will desiccate—burn off—the lesion under locally injected anesthesia. On rare occasion, the person needs the intervention of a subspecialist to perform more extensive removal such as Moh's Chemosurgery, which is a space-age name for a more lengthy but logical procedure. Moh's is a method to remove the skin surrounding the cancer until the microscope reveals no more cancer cells.

The trick is finding a dermatologist who has the time and inclination to visit the home. Most homes are not so fortunate, though I wonder if sometimes it's a lack of effort on the part of the home and its medical director. In any event, the message here from a confirmed nonalarmist is if a bump or lump or "lesion" looks funny and the primary doctor can't give you reassurance that it's absolutely benign, request a dermatologist. You'll be happier in the long run as some of these growths can become disfiguring quickly. By the same token, if a sore on the leg is not responding to basic treatment, it could be a skin cancer masquerading as something else.

Some general surgeons do visit nursing homes and can evaluate surgical issues such as hernias, colostomies, gall bladders, and the like. They also take care of infected boils and some wounds. Many surgeons prefer to see nursing home residents in their offices partly for convenience and partly because they have more equipment available to them there. When a primary-care doctor even *thinks* about a general surgical evaluation, it is usually warranted. The more difficult issues concern wound care and in particular pressure ulcers and vascular ulcers of the legs. I will discuss both these ulcers in chapter 9.

*   *   *

Orthopedic surgeons sometimes have visiting relationships with nursing homes and if not, their office will make arrangements to see the resident in their office. The orthopedist diagnoses and treats fractures and most commonly those are of the shoulder, hip, wrist, and spine. These are the bones that osteoporosis affects the most. People with shoulder, wrist, and hip fractures most often make their way to an emergency room after a fall and may have other trauma such as a head injury.

The best way to prevent hip fractures is through the use of hip protectors. This is a garment that resembles low-profile underwear. In the two side pockets of the underwear nestle hard plastic guards opposite each hip that when worn properly prevent more than 80% of hip fractures. Just for comparison, the two common medications for osteoporosis, alendronate (Fosomax) and risedronate (Actonel), prevent from 0 to 50% of fractures, depending on the study. Another treatment gaining momentum is the use of high-dose cholecalciferol (vitamin D3). Doses of at least 800 to 1000 units per day can prevent not only fractures but falls, too. (There appear to be vitamin D receptors on muscle cells.) Be aware that even though many calcium supplements contain vitamin D, they are usually in lower doses that studies have shown not to be nearly as beneficial. The Evercare program that I mentioned earlier has inaugurated a national campaign that prescribes for its nursing home members a 50,000-unit capsule of vitamin D3 once per month. This is a cheap and easy way to get vitamin D levels up to snuff. It also demonstrates that managed care programs can and do serve a preventive role that ultimately improves the health of its members.

Hip fractures almost always require surgery, except in the rare case of a resident who is approaching her final days or is completely immobile. While it used to be unusual to surgically fix a hip fracture in the elderly, advances in technique and improvement in anesthesia have minimized the trauma and complications of surgery. Leaving a person with an unfixed hip fracture sentences them in most cases to a life of pain. Every move in and out of bed can be unbearable, even with heavy pain meds. I'm not one to give an orthopedist a free pass, but in these situations I've learned almost always to recommend surgery.

I once cared for a resident with severe emphysema and psychiatric problems who had been wasting away and was down to ninety pounds. When she fell and broke her hip, I actually vacillated quite a bit, but in the end just couldn't see recommending surgery. I also thought that she would not cooperate with even a limited physical therapy program after the operation. The rational and reasonable daughter told me she would not be able to live with herself unless she agreed to surgery for her mother, who was also signaling (through her psychotic haze) that she wanted surgery. I gave her almost no chance of surviving and here we are a year later and she is not only alive, but has learned to walk again. I can't say she has the greatest quality of life, but she did return to *her* quality of life.

Shoulder fractures generally do *not* require surgery. If the bones are reasonably aligned after the fracture (what we call a nondisplaced fracture), immobilizing the arm in a sling and swathe will usually heal it. It might take several months and lots of therapy for the shoulder to be functional again and sometimes it never regains the mobility it once had. The sling and swathe apparatus is a sling with a separate strap that goes over and around the back to keep the shoulder and arm from swinging out away from the body. This contraption is hard to put on and many aides and nurses do their best, but without success. If the sling and swathe does not look in the right place or does not hold the arm snugly to the chest, it is not on properly. Appeal to the nurse on duty and if she or he is not sure what to do, be sure the therapist sees your parent soon. Then it is worth raising a *little* Cain and taking this to a more senior nurse so it doesn't happen again.

An important aspect of the care with any fracture is pain control and the doctor needs to be aggressive in giving enough pain medication—usually a narcotic that contains either oxycodone (as in Percocet) or morphine. Codeine (Tylenol #3) and hydrocodone (Vicodin) may not suffice. Be aware that depending on the individual, the narcotic may cause some confusion or grogginess. Patients usually grow tolerant to this side effect and it dissipates in a few days. Others are very sensitive and the doctor needs to reduce the dose to the tiniest one possible. There are some surprising people who have a high pain threshold and really can get by on acetaminophen (Tylenol). See chapter 6 for the lowdown on pain medications.

Wrist fractures are a bit easier in that a cast can be placed that immobilizes the wrist and reduces the pain immediately. The same holds true for fractures that are lower on the leg than the hip, such as the ankle or mid-part (shin) of the lower leg. This assumes that the bones remain in good alignment (are not displaced) and do not require surgery. Many fractures such as rib and spine-vertebral fractures do not require treatment beyond diagnosis. Most fractures heal in about four to six weeks, but the pain and reduced function can take several more weeks to months to improve. While a brace may be easier than a cast, it will not immobilize as well and often falls off.

Some orthopedists are wary of casts for the elderly and for good reason. The cast is very constricting and does not expand if there is swelling. Older people tend to swell more and cannot always signify that they are experiencing pain. I have seen several cases of casts that caused harm by eroding the skin of a swollen wrist or ankle and causing a painful skin sore. The care team may ignore the pain or attribute it to the original fracture. The key point is to refer the person back to the orthopedist immediately if there is any suggestion that a sore under the cast or at the edge of the cast has developed. The orthopedist can easily cut away part of the cast or remove it completely. If there is no sore, the orthopedist can replace the cast and no harm was done. The potential downside to ignoring the problem is a lost limb and we are all familiar with such cases. As a family member, you can ask that the care team examines both exposed ends of the cast several times a week to be sure there are no sores developing—at least in the areas that are visible. When I admit a resident with a cast (or even a long brace for that matter), I include an order to check the skin on a schedule, document any changes, and to call me immediately for any skin breakdown.

There are several new procedures for spine-vertebral fractures. We also call these *compression fractures* and they are the classic osteoporotic fracture often without a known cause. A bad cough, a sneeze, or bending over can cause a compression fracture. The new procedures are known as vertebroplasties and kyphoplasties. They are performed as outpatient procedures (or during a brief hospitalization) involving the injection of a type of bone cement into a fractured and collapsed vertebra of the spine. The theory is that through the injection (and using a balloon to restore proper anatomy in the case of the kyphoplasty) one gives artificial stability to the fracture and thereby reduces the pain. The literature is divided as to when the optimal time for injection is, but the earliest to contemplate would be two to three weeks after fracture and only if the pain is not improving and/or is disabling. While some studies show promising and faster reduction of pain, there have been no randomized controlled trials of this procedure, which is usually the gold standard to prove a treatment's value. Most spinal fractures improve in time with pain medication and/or a back brace. All things being equal, such procedures are usually not performed on frail nursing home residents. Complications occur and include bleeding, infection, leakage of the cement, and clots to the lung.

The other major reason we consult orthopedists is for severe arthritis in a joint such as the knee, which might benefit from an injection of a steroid medication. Some primary-care doctors and most rheumatologists are capable of injecting joints, but if not, an orthopedist would be the ticket.

Urologists deal mainly with plumbing problems in the human urinary system. Kidney doctors address how the kidneys *make* urine while urologists investigate why the urine, once made, is not getting out of the body properly (retention) or is getting out too quickly (incontinence). For retention in men, it's usually a prostate problem and/or a weak bladder. In women, it is usually a bladder issue. A general doctor should be able to evaluate the function of the urinary tract and check for any medications that might be causing a problem. Anticholinergic-containing medications are common in psychiatric medications and cold medications and can cause retention. Severe constipation can push on the bladder and urethra and cause either retention or incontinence.

Many nursing homes have a small portable machine called a bladder scan, which is a type of ultrasound. It measures the amount of urine left in the bladder after the patient urinates (PVR or "post-void residual urine"). Without the machine, the nurse can perform it the old-fashioned way with a catheter. Any amount over 100–150cc for a woman and about 200cc for a man probably necessitates a urologist's visit. The doctors may choose to insert a Foley catheter to allow the bladder to decompress to its normal size again and regain function. Some are in such severe retention they literally have up to 2,000cc (about two quarts) of urine that they cannot empty. This is very uncomfortable and should be easy to recognize in a basic physical exam. Owing to the peculiarities of geriatrics, retention even this massive is missed now and then.

Some urologists also can help with the evaluation and treatment of incontinence. A full discussion of incontinence is beyond the scope of this book but visit the National Association for Continence website at www.nafc.org. It will tell you more than you might ever need to know about the urinary system. Most urologists can evaluate the urinary system noninvasively, but occasionally— with severe retention or recurrent blood in the urine—they will perform a cystoscopy. Some do this under local anesthesia in their office and others only in a surgi-center with more serious anesthesia. The urologist or general doctor may prescribe medications that slow down the overactive bladder such as tolterodine (Detrol) or oxybutynin (Ditropan) or make the urethra a bit wider such as terazocin (Hytrin) or tamsulosin (Flomax). No matter what they try, these medications work less well in the frail elderly and often make no functional difference at all. The staff still has to use adult diapers and take the resident to the toilet every two hours on a so-called toileting program. If the medications don't work, have them stopped. They can cause dry mouth, which paradoxically increases thirst and aggravates the incontinence.

Elevated PSA (prostate-specific antigen, which *can* be a marker for cancer of the prostate) levels are more a concern of free-living adult males. The official recommendations are that unless the patient has at least ten years life expectancy, we don't perform screening PSAs. By the way, for mammograms in elderly women, we stop when there are five years or less life expectancy.

Otolaryngologists or ENTs (ear, nose, and throat doctors) generally serve two or three roles in a nursing home population. They are great at cleaning out ears that for some reason the regular physician cannot. Some earwax has been embedded in the ear canal for years and even bleeds when it is dislodged. Many a hearing aid has been avoided by a good cleaning of the ears. I once disimpacted the ears of a 102-year-old man of quite a bit of wax. It looked like it had been there forever, and when I asked him, he said the last time he cleaned out his ears was on the eve of World War II! He was able to communicate much more freely after all the wax was removed and it was gratifying to have helped him. ENTs also are knowledgeable about tracheostomy care. Most residents with trachs run into problems with them. There are different fittings and different types of trachs depending on whether the person eats or wishes to speak through the trach. A good ENT may be hard to have visit the home, but some therapy agencies provide a onetime consultation from a respiratory therapist that may be as good.

All the Other "-Ologists"

Neurologists sometimes come into the nursing home, but mostly we send residents out to their offices. The most common reason that I use a neurologist is to help with management of Parkinson's disease. Like diabetes, this field has gone from relatively simple to complex. Most of the medications work to increase the amount of L-dopa in the brain but in different ways. The medications are often used to complement each other and can also cause significant side effects that include low blood pressure, nausea, and abnormal movements called dyskinesias. These are abnormal "jerky" movements with which the world has become familiar through the actor Michael J. Fox. Generally, overdosage of L-dopa causes dyskinesias but many patients tolerate these movements as the price they must pay to free up their muscles from the imprisoning stiffness of Parkinson's.

Another compelling reason to consult a neurologist is when one is not even sure a tremor or stiffness *is* from Parkinson's. There are no lab tests or X-rays that will diagnose Parkinson's with certainty. There are other causes of tremors, such as essential tremor (aka benign or senile—think Katharine Hepburn), overactive thyroid, and more serious brain diseases. Medications like the antipsychotics (especially the older ones like haloperidol—Haldol) have been known to cause tremors. A good neurologist can ferret out the possible causes and might even save your parent from the side effects of some of these drugs. I will say that the older one *is*, the less typical the signs of Parkinson's can be and sometimes a trial of anti-Parkinson's medications is the only way to discern the diagnosis. If these medications have not helped in a significant and functional way, ask the doctors to stop them.

As we already discussed, the behavioral symptoms of dementia are usually not the province of the neurologist, and onset of dementia generally occurs prior to admission. I occasionally call a neurologist for issues related to seizures and if it's safe to take someone off an antiseizure medication. You may be wondering why stop a seizure medication? Aren't they preventing dangerous seizures in the first place? Some are started with little hard evidence that a seizure really took place. Some were started preventively in patients with brain surgery, brain trauma, or a tumor. Most are sedating and many have side effects. Some of our best work is done in the less is more vein, and eliminating unnecessary medications can be salutary.

Cardiologists prove useful for very complex congestive heart failure though most heart failure is bread and butter, so to speak, and well within the province of a primary-care doctor. If the doctor feels a confirmatory evaluation is needed, so be it, but there is little benefit from regular trips back and forth to the cardiologist. Heart rhythm abnormalities are another story. Most primary-care folks can care for the irregular atrial fibrillation rhythm about which we spoke in the section on blood thinners and heart medications in the previous chapter. Someone with an exceedingly slow rhythm (bradycardia) and who has symptoms of fainting or light-headedness should see a cardiologist to be sure a pacemaker is not needed. This assumes a few things. First, the primary physician reviewed the list of medications to be sure that the culprit is not merely a medication—like beta-blockers and calcium-channel blockers—that slows the heartbeat. Reducing or stopping these drugs can bring the heartbeat to normal and cure the problem. Even some older glaucoma drops that have beta-blocking activity (Timolol comes to mind) have been known to slow the heartbeat. Second, does your parent's life trajectory warrant the intervention of a pacemaker?

Many families of my patients have made the courageous decision that the burden of living may be greater than the benefit. This also arises when a pacemaker battery reaches the end of its life (usually around ten years after implanting it). The family of one of my residents has chosen not to replace the battery in their mom, who is severely demented and can no longer speak or recognize her family members. If that is the case, I avoid even *bringing in* a cardiologist. They have a funny way of even inadvertently talking a family member into the operation to change a battery. Again, don't let anyone tell you that you *have to* do something; in caring for the frail elderly, there are no absolutes.

Lung doctors or pulmonologists are rarely needed except in the occasional case that the doctor can't determine if the breathing problem is the heart or the lungs. A person with a lung tumor or shadow seen on an X-ray may benefit from an opinion but only if you really plan to *do* something about it. Why put your parent through an invasive bronchoscopy (slipping a fiber-optic tube into the windpipe and lungs to have a look, under some type of anesthesia) or extensive CT scan if she is so frail and close to the end of her life that you would not contemplate surgery anyway? These are person-by-person calculations but what you *must* ask the specialist or primary physician who recommends further testing is: 1) What will we *do* with the information gained by this test? and 2) Do we *need* to do anything? You might even ask that age-old question, "If it was your mom, Doc, what would you do?" If the "doc" hesitates or says something like, "Well, it's really your decision," you should assume that a viable alternative is to say no or that you could wait and not rush. Again, *there are no musts*.

Skin testing for tuberculosis raises many questions. The vast majority of residents either has a negative test or has a long history of a positive test and does not need it repeated. A positive test means that at some point in their life they were "infected" with tuberculosis bacteria. The body was able to establish a firewall through its normal defenses and neutralize the "infection." The danger is that late in life, when the immune system is weakened either naturally or via medications (usually steroids like Prednisone), the tuberculosis can reactivate and cause full-blown disease. There is also an intermediate group of residents whose skin test *recently* converted to positive from a known prior negative. Lung specialists often have strong opinions on this score and it might be reasonable to bring one into the discussion early. The prophylactic treatment is usually a medication called isoniazid (INH), which is taken once a day for about six to nine months. The older the patient, the more likely the side effect of liver damage from this medication. The pulmonologist can be helpful in thinking through these complicated decisions.

Stomach specialists (gastroenterologists) are occasionally asked for an opinion regarding internal bleeding. Sometimes the brisk-ness of the bleeding (falling blood counts, black stools, vomiting blood) biases the medical team toward hospitalizing the resident. All things being equal, this is not a bad, idea, as the resident often needs blood transfusions and close monitoring. I have found that even if a living will and prior conversation with family seem to pre-clude hospitalization, staff and family are uncomfortable allowing someone possibly to bleed to death. What they don't understand is that most internal bleeding is self-limited and stops by itself. More often than not, the bleeding is slow and the gastroenterologist can render an opinion about choices for treatment.

Again, ask the same questions raised earlier. If the blood counts are stable and your parent is not bothered by any symptoms, is any further testing necessary? The further testing in these cases usually involves a scoping of the lower or upper tracts or both. While these are easier procedures than they used to be, endoscopy is still inva-sive. It may turn up a cancer or tumor that you would choose not to do anything about anyway, especially if the resident's quality of life is not great to start with. I have had many alert patients who are capable of calling their own shots refuse endoscopy and are none the worse for it. Many of the gastroenterologists with whom I work, to their credit, would not even recommend endoscopy on a frail nursing home resident with dementia. While I hesitate to mention it, though, there are some few who know they benefit financially from performing procedures and will never present the option of observation over invasion.

Artificial feeding tubes (or PEGs for percutaneous endoscopic gastrostomy tubes) are devices that are implanted through the abdominal wall directly into the stomach in order to deliver liquid feedings. I will address the ethical pros and cons of these tubes in chapter 12, but suffice it to say that a gastroenterologist is the one who performs placement of these tubes. I have in recent memory encountered only one gastroenterologist who questioned the ethics of placing a tube so don't rely on him or her to be a moral sounding board. When it comes to these tubes, many are technicians—guns for hire, or whatever you wish to call them. After a tube is placed, they usually last about six to nine months and then need to be replaced. Because of the type of the original tube, a gastroenterology specialist best handles these replacements, though I suppose in some locales surgeons might do them as well. The doctor requesting the change should ask for a balloon-type tube as a replacement. That way, when it needs to be changed again (and these wear out a bit faster) the primary physician can do it at the bedside.

In some nursing homes, nurses are allowed by policy to replace the tubes, but usually this is in an emergent situation when the tube falls out by itself. The danger of leaving it out for more than about twelve hours is that the tract through which the tube enters the stomach can close up. This would mean a second invasive procedure rather than a simple bedside procedure. That is why the nurses in some homes replace the tube with a temporary tube until the physician can replace it with an appropriate tube.

Before you even go the route of considering a feeding tube, the gastroenterologist may help uncover why a patient has stopped eating or is losing weight. Most internists and family medicine doctors should be able to initiate this evaluation as well. The causes of anorexia (loss of appetite) are legion. Several medications, including those that act against Alzheimer's, Parkinson's, and depression, can cause loss of appetite. Digoxin at too high a level can do the same. Ill-fitting dentures, a yeast infection of the mouth known as thrush, and stomach ailments such as peptic ulcers, bowel obstructions, acid reflux, and constipation may result in weight loss. Severe constipation that results in hard balls of stool can block the rectum (known as fecal impaction). This is often hinted at by a nasty smell in the room and an abdomen that feels tight and distended. The patient may even vomit material that smells like stool. The nursing assistants may report poor or no bowel movements for several days to a week or more. Sometimes paradoxically they can report daily bowel movements or even loose movements and throw the care team off the track. It behooves any physician evaluating significant anorexia and weight loss to perform a simple rectal exam. It can reveal blood in the stool (sometimes a sign of colon cancer) or an impaction that otherwise was missed.

I have relieved many a patient over the years by manually "disimpacting" them of stool. It's not pretty and it's not comfortable for anyone. Nursing homes are sometimes reluctant to even check for an impaction because they can be cited by the state for a so-called "sentinel" event—i.e., an event that should never occur. This is one of the most asinine elements of the survey process. In the best of all worlds, impactions should *not* occur but they *do*. By making the homes afraid to report them, the surveying teams are hurting our nursing home residents. Some physicians are not on-site enough to disimpact or to take that level of interest in their residents. In these cases, if there is a hint of an impaction, ask the nurse if she can check the rectum. Otherwise, beg for a gastroenterologist to pay a visit.

If none of these leads pay off, we are left with the possibilities of depression or advanced dementia. The former is treatable but difficult to diagnose in residents with complicating dementia. It is *sometimes* worth a trial of an antidepressant or, less often, an appetite stimulant (see chapter 6). It also is worth checking a set of labs to exclude a metabolic issue or dehydration as the cause (though it can also be the result) of the appetite loss. The specter of cancer always looms in the discussion of weight loss, but a fairly limited examination and simple blood tests can usually exclude this. In my experience with nursing home patients, advanced dementia is a much more common cause of weight loss and dehydration.

The last major reason to call in a gastroenterologist is for a resident with diarrhea that doesn't seem to want to quit. There are some obvious causes for diarrhea in a nursing home resident and most primary-care doctors can get the ball rolling on an evaluation. Often the resident is ingesting too many prescribed laxatives, the diarrhea is a side effect of another medication, or—if the resident is on artificial feedings—the rate or type of feeding needs adjusting. A major cause is an infection known as "C. diff," which I will address in chapter 11. If the diarrhea persists despite these considerations, a specialist is entirely appropriate.

Kidney specialists, or nephrologists, rarely come into a home to see patients. On the occasions that residents need their help, they will usually need to see them in the office setting. In the last chapter, we discussed medications to treat anemia and calcium balance for impending renal failure. These medications are perhaps best prescribed in consultation with a nephrologist. There are parts of the country without easy access to these specialists. In these circumstances, the primary-care doctor is well versed enough to undertake this him- or herself.

As the function of the kidney declines to a clearance of 10–15cc per minute (or the creatinine rises to well above four or five), the question of dialysis sometimes arises. There are many cultural and geographic issues at play here. Many (most?) families rightly see dialysis as a heroic measure that their loved one would wish to forego. It takes a great deal of cooperation and mental alertness to participate in the twice or thrice weekly four- to five-hour sessions, not to mention the transportation to and fro. Add to that a problem with what we call "access" and one has the recipe for a potential disaster.

"Access" refers to the need to *access* the vascular system in order to draw off blood, cleanse it in the dialysis machine, and return it to the body. In younger people, access is achieved through a "graft" or "fistula," which is a surgically created conduit of a major artery to a vein in the arm that then remains under the skin. In older people these are harder to create and maintain. Most access in the frail elderly is achieved though a device called a Permacath. This is a tube or catheter that a surgeon places during a surgical procedure. There are risks to the placement, and once implanted it can become the focus of infection and bleeding. Even more important, it can be annoying and the external part hangs outside the body near the clavicle and upper chest area. It can be wrapped in gauze, but the person must be aware enough not to fiddle with the line and certainly not to try to pull it out. *Perma*cath is a bit of a misnomer since most run into complications and need to be changed within a year. Sometimes infections of the catheter require this and sometimes they are beset with blood clots that render them unusable. These are among the many reasons that dialysis is usually not feasible for someone who is frail or has dementia.

Like the gastroenterologist not discussing the ethics of feeding tubes, kidney specialists sometimes will refrain from that discussion on dialysis as well. Even when a kidney specialist recommends dialysis it is not always a slam dunk that the person needs it. I used to care for a resident who had been talked into dialysis and suffered through it for about a year until she decided that it was no longer for her. She was told by the kidney specialist that by foregoing it she would soon die and that she should go on hospice. About two years later, still very much alive and very much off dialysis, hospice decided she was not in fact dying and "graduated" her. About another year after that and after developing dementia, she finally succumbed. What did all this mean? By the lab numbers, she certainly appeared to need dialysis, but appearances can be deceiving. Choosing against dialysis for ethical reasons or simply not wishing to live that kind of life does not always equate to ending it.

In contrast, I do have *one* patient in a nursing home who has been on dialysis for several years and seems to have a decent quality of life. He was an exceptionally intelligent, determined, and persuasive man (a clergyman, in fact) his whole life, and the ups and downs of dialysis—he has had many of them—have not fazed him. I have to regard him as the exception, but he has taught me that each person is unique—I need to approach the decision for or against dialysis individually. Ask the specialist for his opinion, but also ask what other options exist and remember that the decision is yours and your loved one's.

I think you can see that specialists are a mixed blessing. Part of my frustration is with our health care system that values specialists over generalists. It is also failing to train the next generation of generalists (and as far as geriatricians go, *fuggedaboudit*) who are confident enough in their skills to forego the need for too many specialists. There are times when a primary-care doctor needs help and I hope I have characterized those periods for you. Do not neglect your gut feelings, though, when it comes to recommendations for interventions with lifelong implications, such as feeding tubes and dialysis. Because a specialist recommends a treatment doesn't mean it's right for your loved one. As the saying goes, "If you call a plumber, he'll fix the pipes." Think about what your parent would say if he or she could. You must be her substitute and, many times, child knows best!

8

Psychiatrists and Psychologists: Why Are They So Busy?

The busiest consultants in our home are the geriatric psychiatrists, followed closely by their colleagues, the geriatric psychologists. In the prior chapters regarding medications and consultants, I explored many of the concerns about mental disease in the nursing home. Whether it's depression, dementia, or dysthymia, one has to ask if the burden of these problems is comparable to the general geriatric population, and the answer is a resounding no. Many residents of nursing homes come from families who have tried desperately to keep them at home for as long as possible. But nursing homes are institutions, too, and as such end up housing people that are left behind by the rest of society.

Many of the residents of the homes in which I have worked have had enough psychological, behavioral, and social problems over the years that they have burned out their families. That is not always the case, but it is true *enough* of our time that it gives nursing homes a different flavor these days. New York and other states are experiencing an interesting phenomenon, which could be called the "ungraying" of nursing homes. State governments are asking more homes to help house those suffering from serious mental illnesses and substance abuse. Many of these people had been hospitalized in the equivalent of state hospitals, some had been homeless, and many simply can't live on their own. Some have suffered trauma during a fight or accident. *The New York Times* recently described one publicly funded home on Long Island with a particularly young population in which drug sales, addiction, and even prostitution was widespread.

These homes are still the exception, but elements of these changes can be witnessed in most homes. Our home admitted a woman in her midforties with multiple medical conditions but also significant mental issues. When she was presented to us for admission, the community people seeking to have her admitted either downplayed her abnormal behaviors or we overlooked some of them. When a home's beds are not filled, it tends to be more liberal admitting people it might on another day decline. Though we clearly have standards and by law should not admit someone for whom we cannot care, we thought with a good psychiatrist on board and a great staff, we would manage and even do right by this hard-luck case. We could not have been more wrong, and by the end of almost a year with us, she had alienated the entire staff and, more significantly, compromised the quality of life of our other residents. When we finally corralled her family, they did admit that she had been diagnosed years ago with paranoid schizophrenia and antisocial personality disorder that had mostly gone untreated.

Once someone like this resident is admitted, it is very hard to transfer her elsewhere. The mental health infrastructure in this country is so damaged that inpatient care is only available for the most dangerous and the most delusional. She finally ended up being committed short-term after countless efforts and then signed out to live on the street again. What does help a home deal with these issues is if enough families complain and raise a ruckus. Even a call to the ombudsman may give the home enough ammunition to attempt a change. We have occasionally called the ombudsman ourselves!

There are other situations in which an elderly person, who may have been calm enough on admission, develops dangerous behaviors due to progression of dementia. Treatment modalities were discussed earlier and psychiatrists, psychologists, and medications may provide some help. In the end, though, many residents should be on nursing units that can expect and handle these behaviors (hitting, biting, and sexual aggression). The decision that a home cannot continue to house such a person is fraught with difficulties and is never made lightly. Sometimes a special dementia unit, utilizing creative behavioral approaches, can address the issue and the abnormal behaviors settle down. Other times, one needs to seek a change for the safety of the other residents and staff.

The home should be familiar with local alternatives. Our own local hospitals have fewer and fewer inpatient psychiatric beds, and they dislike admitting people with dementia who may be incontinent and have medical challenges to boot. These inpatient units tend to have younger patients with pure psychiatric problems, and our nursing home residents really do change the milieu for the worse. When we send our residents to the ER for evaluation, they are almost always sent back to us within twelve hours. They are deemed either not a danger to themselves or others (our residents often mysteriously calm down in ERs) or are treated with sedatives and sent right back. The ERs don't always grasp that sedation is a short-term fix, not very safe, and not the way we are supposed to be caring for these souls.

We sometimes have luck by establishing a relationship with a particular psychiatrist who will admit the resident at least for a few days and treat them, but again this usually involves heavy sedatives. We have to promise that we will take the resident back so that the patient does not become the hospital's headache to find another setting for (known as a "placement problem"). The truth is there is *no* good place for them and only rarely is the hospital or anyone able to secure a long-term bed in a psychiatric facility. Some of these facilities are state-run and have checkered reputations that—being composed entirely of those with severe behavioral issues—one would expect. But that's a problem for the policy makers and health planners.

The Depression Epidemic

Never underestimate the importance and dangers of depression in the elderly. One of my most important teaching moments came about ten years ago. I was at the home early one morning to make rounds. The nurses had left me a message about one of my favorite residents, who I will call Bernie. Bernie was a man of irrepressible charm and panache. Though he was severely disabled by Parkinson's disease and other maladies, he had a permanent smile creased across his face and loved regaling us with stories of his youth. He had been a star athlete in school and had pictures to prove it. He was much loved by his family, and though he had been widowed some time ago, he had dated following his wife's death.

The reason the nurses wanted me to see him, or so they

explained in the brief note, was that "Bernie has been talking about life not being worth living." I must have been in a hurry to get to the hospital or another home, I'm not sure which, but I made one of those rough calculations and thought I could safely move this down low on my triage list or even handle it the next day. Bernie was so weak and dependent that he would never be physically capable of hurting himself. Besides, that couldn't be *my* Bernie. If anyone had gotten to the last of Erik Erikson's stages of life and found it to be full of "integrity," it was Bernie.

I went on my merry way, saw some really "sick" residents, made hospital rounds, did some paperwork, and went home that night. Around seven the next morning, while on my way to the nursing home, I received a page on my beeper marked "urgent." I called in and the nurse in charge told me to get there in a hurry, they had found Bernie with a cord around his neck. I sped the last mile, ran to the building, and saw Bernie in bed, blue as cobalt, the removed electrical cord dangling nearby. He was taking some difficult, labored breaths, but the oxygen the nurse had placed was already beginning to help him. Thankfully, by the time the EMTs arrived, Bernie's color had improved and he was beginning to talk. Bernie survived and was hospitalized on a psychiatric unit for a suicide attempt.

Why did he try to kill himself? Bernie had become entangled in a love triangle at the home. He had recently attended a reminiscence group and recognized one of the women as someone he had courted about sixty-five years before, in high school. He tried at the nursing home to rekindle the romance but she was seeing another resident. Whatever integrity Bernie had banked turned to despair and he made the comment to the nurses about life not being worth living. Whether this was true depression or a plea for help was immaterial; I should have checked it out pronto. We were taught in my geriatrics training that elderly white males have the highest suicide rate after young adults, but somehow that didn't seem to fit Bernie.

Bernie recovered nicely and went on to live a reasonable life back at the home. He eventually died of something else, but the image of him, the would-be suicide with the smile across his face, was imprinted on me. I take any threat seriously enough to evaluate it myself or make sure another physician does so in a hurry. This is, in part, why psychiatrists and psychologists in nursing homes are so busy. Thinking, aware elders can arguably see every day as judgment day—the day they weigh, after a very long life, whether they are basking in integrity or suffering in despair. Add to this the burden of psychiatric symptoms that accompany dementia, and you can see why most residents of nursing homes at some point come face-to-face with a mental health worker.

Bernie's love triangle astounded me. How often do we think of our parents and grandparents as fossilized, chaste, and prudish creatures of another age? The shock to us is that they, too, led lives of passion and love. They just didn't talk about it and perhaps that's why the sadness and depression and disappointment spill over late in life.

When I was a resident in training in Boston, I took care of a ninety-year-old woman, who I will call Margaret, from a large rough-and-tumble South Boston Irish family. I would see her every few months for a blood pressure check, but otherwise she was healthy. Margaret was the quiet matriarch type, almost shy, and very prim. Then one day after I had not seen her for about half a year, one of her granddaughters brought her to the clinic. Margaret had lost thirty pounds, was barely speaking, and appeared pensive and withdrawn. I did the basic exam and a few tests to confirm that there was nothing physically wrong with her.

On the next visit a few days later, I asked the family (now there were several grandchildren in tow) to leave the room. I asked her if there was anything else she wanted to tell me. While wringing her hands, she stated that when she was nineteen years old, she had become pregnant and had had an abortion. She later married someone else and settled in to her life but always felt guilty about the affair and the baby she had aborted. Suddenly, at age ninety, she could literally not live with herself. She wanted to share this with her family and wanted me to chair the session. I don't recall if I had anyone more senior from the medical staff join us, but I called the family back in and she told them in muted tones what she had told me. Jaws dropped, tears flowed, minds expanded, and our job was now to get her better. The family, despite profound shock, could not have been more empathetic and helpful.

Margaret did not respond to psychiatric treatment or medication and ended up being one of my few patients to undergo electric shock treatment. She became confused and delirious with the treatment that was done in the hospital over the course of two weeks. She gradually improved and was able to gain some weight and stop ruminating about her guilt. I was at that point close to finishing my residency and passed her along to the incoming class of interns. I'm not sure what became of her, but like Bernie, Margaret's situation taught me about depression in the elderly.

This case also raises the question of so-called ECT (electroconvulsive therapy) in the elderly. Since Margaret, I have had a handful of patients undergo this treatment. Our images of this stem partly from One Flew Over the Cuckoo's Nest, in which the images of the ECT-induced seizures were heart stopping. Since then, the field has changed quite a bit and—through technological advances, better anesthesia, and treatment to only one side of the brain at a time (unipolar treatment)—is much safer. Whether it is effective is a very difficult question to answer. I have read several review articles on the matter. They agree that there have been only three or four randomized controlled studies of ECT in the elderly in the last twenty-five years. Some of the reviews found each of these studies to be flawed and others found them acceptable. Some reviews found no support for ECT and others claimed both support and safety. The jury is clearly out and we may never have an answer, but sometimes our hand is forced.

Bernie, who did not undergo ECT, and Margaret, who did, would be the types of older people who are candidates for this controversial treatment. The more one suffers from dementia, the more pervasive the confusion from ECT, and the harder it is to peer through the haze to glimpse if the treatment is helping. We reserve ECT in the elderly for people who are literally dying from depression. This almost always involves severe loss of appetite and weight loss despite treatment with antidepressants and talk therapy. The literature and research do reveal enough *individual* success stories to make it an option under these circumstances. I even had one resident who had a series of treatments and then underwent what was called maintenance therapy of ECT about every month as an outpatient. Some families are unalterably opposed to ECT on humanitarian grounds, though most will be willing to try it if all else fails.

Your Right to Know

Let's touch on a few other issues in regard to psychiatrists and psychologists. Is it fair to expect the home or primary-care doctor to tell you (or your loved one) in advance that a psychiatrist is coming? As a general principle, a nursing home *should* inform you whenever it calls in a consultant. First, you deserve to know and want to know that your parent has developed a condition that is beyond the ken and expertise of the regular staff. Second, you will most likely be seeing a bill from the consultant and may need to pay all or part of it as a copay or deductible. Third, the consultant may need to perform a procedure (such as a dermatologist removing a growth) and may need to receive consent from the family. We have fielded not a few angry calls from families who mostly were upset that they were left out of the equation. We then "required" that the physician or someone else notify the family. In practice, if a resident goes out of the building to visit a specialist, our scheduler has to notify the family to inquire about transportation requirements. If the specialist comes to our home, the onus is on us to let the family know.

In reality this is easier said than done. We're doing better than we used to, but we are not perfect. In the case of mental health visits, families really *must* be in the loop. A decent psychiatrist or psychologist will want to talk to the family to learn more history about the problem. More often than not, there is prior history when it comes to depression.

If the psychiatrist prescribes psychoactive medications, he or she needs to explain the rationale and potential side effects. As I discussed earlier, the antipsychotic medications carry so-called "black box" warnings and families really need to hear this. Most of the professionals with whom I have worked *do* contact families or at least leave a message. However, some years ago I interviewed a potential psychiatrist for our home who told me he *didn't* talk to families because it "took too much time." I escorted him out of the building, but it gave me the sense there are more out there like him.

You should definitely 'fess up to the consultant if there are any skeletons lurking in your or your loved one's closet. You might even provide names of prior therapists. They may know what treatment worked best in the past. If the psychiatrist is there because your parent threatened to kill herself, it is germane that she has threatened this for sixty-plus years just to get attention. Perhaps the home *is* overreacting by transferring her out to the local psychiatric inpatient unit. Most psychiatrists have to make these judgments every day and are comfortable documenting their rationale in the chart. This protects the home and saves your parent from an unnecessary transfer

Gentle Reminders and Keeping Track

One other point about psychiatrists in particular (and all consultants in general): They may need several reminders to actually show up at the home. They often receive the initial request by cell phone, pager, carrier pigeon, or smoke signal and messages often become lost. A conscientious medical director has ways of keeping track, but you would be surprised how often things fall between the cracks. Even when the specialist comes quickly, his assessment may be buried among other papers or filed incorrectly and the recommendations are never endorsed. One of my primary-care physicians was away recently and asked me to cover another unit at our home. To my dismay, I found that there were actually two clipboards in circulation and some of the nurses and clerks put consultations on one clipboard and some on the other. The nurse manager and physician were only aware that one clipboard existed. I hope I'm not airing our dirty laundry by telling you that the parallel universe clipboard contained information from four months before that our physician had never examined. Thankfully, nothing crucial was missed, which also makes you wonder what the heck all these consultations were good for; but as they say, let's not go there. Our nursing home is relatively well organized and this was a great doctor and a great nurse. I think you get my drift. Much like my advice on tracking down the medication list from the hospital and taking it yourself to the home at the time of transfer, you must keep track of any consultant visits and be sure their opinions are acted upon. You should also let your doctor know from the get-go if you want to be notified of any consultations. If you wish to add to that notification for any change in medication, you can do that, too. Sometimes the best person to help you with that is the social worker or nurse manager, who can tape a statement to that effect to the front of the chart.

The "Difficult" Patient: An Accident Waiting to Happen?

Lastly, I want to talk about the resident who is adamantly refusing to play ball. I'm sure this resonates with some of you. You may have been in the situation where a hospitalization was precipitated by some crisis—like a fall, a broken hip, or pneumonia. Your parent was the proverbial accident waiting to happen and it was almost a blessing in disguise that she needed to be admitted and then transferred to a nursing home for rehabilitation. Now you can't *imagine* her going home. The risk for another injury is great and the hard-won peace of mind you have with her in the home will be lost in an instant if she returns home. But she won't listen to reason and every visit or call echoes with the drumbeat of "Take me out of this place, now!"

Your first move is to rely on the advice of the experts at the home. Is it really unsafe or could she possibly live in an assisted living facility or at home with help? The social worker, physician, and above all the physical/occupational therapist will give you the best guidance. If you don't feel they are adequate or you just want another opinion, hire a geriatric manager to come in for a onetime visit. Once you know what's safe and what's in her best interest, you will be more sure of your decision. Don't forget that in this equation, you are at least as important a variable as your parent. The analogy to pediatrics is obvious. In taking care of kids, the parent is as much a part of the treatment plan as the child. In geriatrics, the child is as much a part of the management plan as the parent.

Each family and each set of family relationships is different. There are some residents of nursing homes who were not blue-ribbon parents and their children will not bend over backward to accommodate their desires. There are others who were the Michael Jordans of parenting and the kids can never do enough or sacrifice enough in return. Just know that if you are in the latter school, your Herculean efforts may well take away from either you or your own kids. The "sandwich generation" can get eaten alive, so be careful. If this makes no sense to you, consider getting a therapist of your own to help sort it out. Whenever I've recommended that to sons and daughters in need, they've never been sorry.

Also remember that behaviors and statements by your parent don't exist in a vacuum. If you think back, she may have reacted to any change in her life in a negative, pessimistic way. I have a resident right now in the nursing home who laces every exchange with anyone who will listen with pleas to go home. Her loving and long-suffering family tells me horror stories of her being at home even with full-time help. Her medical needs are too great for assisted living and she really *is* in the right place. Though she is quite aware most of the time, she does not back up her regressed behavior with any concrete plan to "spring" herself. The fact that she cannot formulate a plan means: a) though aware, she cannot climb to the next level of understanding risks and benefits; and b) she likely realizes that she has no alternative but to stay.

Though it may sound cruel, let the ravings go on. It may be your parent's last defense and exactly what is getting her through each day. If you can't take it, then visit less often or put your answering machine on. There will come a time when you can resume being a constant and dutiful child, but these transitions are the hardest. When someone coined the phrase "old age isn't for sissies" they may have had the child as much in mind as the parent. "Childing" is indeed tough stuff and no one should underestimate it.

If your parent is cognizant enough to wage a practical or legal challenge, that *could* change the equation. It still does not make her competent in a legal sense and you may have to go the formal and expensive legal route of declaring her incompetent and in need of a guardian such as yourself. On the other hand, a judge may find her competent and able to make these decisions and arrangements for herself. The courts usually ask for two doctors' opinions as to competence: These do not need to be psychiatrists, though many times they are. The most recent trend is for a judge to parse the issue and find the resident is able to make decisions in certain spheres, like health, but not in others, such as financial planning or living arrangements. In these nettlesome and heartrending situations, it helps to have the facility's psychologist see your parent as an objective party and provide tools for your parent to begin to build a new life at the nursing home and not to constantly look back. A parting piece of advice: Don't let yourself be held hostage by a rigid and unrealistic parent. You can still love him or her, but love yourself and your own kids, too.

9

To Hospitalize or Not to Hospitalize

There is an old saying: A nursing home is no place for a sick person. In many parts of the country the slightest cough or fever still prompts physicians to order (by phone in some cases and without laying eyes on the patient) a hospital transfer and admission. Well, the old maxim may need to be turned on its head since these days a *hospital* is no place for a sick person. And the hospital is especially no place for an *old* and *frail* sick person. Infections abound, restraints and catheters are used too freely, and the hospital staff seems to react in horror that it has to care for a person of advanced years. To some extent the hospitals are right: Nursing homes can and do take care of sick people. Why should a hospital keep a forty-five-year-old with a massive heart attack waiting in the ER on a stretcher for a bed when the ninety-nine-year-old upstairs with pneumonia could as easily be treated in the nursing home? Let's talk about the pros and cons of hospitalizing a frail nursing home resident.

Actual hands-on care differs in the makeup of the staff. The hospital care is nurse-driven whereas nurses and nursing assistants drive nursing home care. Nurses are skilled at assessing conditions and changes in condition, enacting care plans, passing medications, dressing wounds, and more. On top of that, they have inordinate amounts of paperwork, which takes them away from the bedside. There are very few nursing assistants on an acute inpatient hospital unit and some are lucky to have even one. A single nursing assistant cannot possibly do all the personal care on all the patients, so either the work is shunted to the nurse or it just does not get done. It used to be the province of the nurse to make beds, change bedpans, get the patients up out of bed, and feed them if they need help. I'm told in the old days nurses even gave massages! With the hurly-burly nature of hospitals these days, the nurses simply cannot begin to complete these tasks.

The two main care items that are lost in the shuffle are getting people out of bed and feeding them while out of bed. It is not unusual for a patient of mine to spend seven days in the hospital and never once be helped out of bed. For the relatively young nursing home resident that can actually stand, this is less of a problem; the nurses tend to get them up to a chair. I know most of my patients are not easy and take extra work to get out of bed. They are no easier in the nursing home yet we get 298 out of 300 people out of bed every day and sometimes twice a day. The only two who *don't* get out of bed *won't* get out of bed because they choose not to.

Staying in bed is the direct cause of the bedsores that one often sees on residents returning from the hospital. I have had residents in our home for five years who go to the hospital and develop their first bedsore within three days. The cruel irony of this is that by letting the patient wallow in bed, the nurses cannot even check the skin that carefully; the bedsore is missed until we readmit them to the nursing home. Were it not that we perform and document a careful skin check on their return, for all the world it looks like the bedsore began on our watch. We recently started a wound-care team to review our residents with wounds and confirmed that 80–90% of our bedsores started elsewhere.

I also have a pet peeve concerning how the nurses try to feed my patients in the hospital. Almost uniformly when I go to visit, I see my patient propped up on pillows at a forty-five-degree angle at best with the food tray on a table in front of them and out of reach. In many cases, no one has opened the plastic-wrapped food or helped them eat. I challenge anyone to swallow in that position and not choke. I have tried it and it's darn hard. Fluids are even worse, and downright dangerous. The slippery slope then begins. Nurse finds tray not eaten, reports patient as consuming 10% of tray. Doctor made aware, orders nutritionist consultation that further documents and memorializes "poor intake." GI specialist called in who recommends permanent feeding tube through wall of stomach while mumbling something like, "You can't let your mother starve to death." I hate to be harsh, but I've seen it so many times that it would be laughable if it weren't so tragic.

Advantages of Treating in Place

At our home and at most nursing homes, besides getting the resident out of bed, we create a dining environment that is social and conducive to eating. We also hire "feeders" who directly assist or feed our less independent people. When that's not enough, the social workers, nursing staff, and activities folks all chip in and do what needs to be done.

What about the notion that only hospitals have the technology and equipment to take care of acutely ill people? Due to the advent of sub-acute care, nursing homes have had to reinvent themselves. Facilities like ours are now capable of starting and/or completing a course of intravenous antibiotics. Most homes have nurses or a contract with an outside service that can begin and maintain intravenous lines. We have available to us any antibiotic or intravenous medication that can be offered in a hospital. The occasional exception to this is inherent in the costliness of some of these medications that I addressed in chapter 4. We perform sophisticated wound care either on our own or continue what started in the hospital.

Nursing homes have, by necessity, become comfortable with the use of techniques and tests that hospitals traditionally utilize. If a resident becomes dehydrated, we even have an alternative to intravenous fluids called dermatoclysis (clysis for short). This is a means of giving fluid through the fatty layers of the body under the skin known as subcutaneous tissue. It works surprisingly well and avoids the need to keep restarting an intravenous. An intravenous is precariously placed in a vein and if the resident moves the wrong way, it can easily be dislodged. The intravenous is also more irksome because it resides in the arm and limits the movement of that limb. We are loath to use restraints to keep the intravenous in place; the clysis is preferable. We place the small needle in the wall of the abdomen or the thigh and change the site every few days. The resident generally does not even know it's there. The major limitation is that we cannot give fluid as quickly with a clysis as with an intravenous, but this is only an issue with severe low blood pressure, such as occurs with a major intestinal bleed.

Another sea change is the availability of different kinds of services in long-term care that were not previously accessible. We can order any blood test and have the results the same day in most cases. In our home, the laboratory that we use supplies a phlebotomy service that arrives at seven A.M. every day. If, in the afternoon, we need a test emergently, the service will come back to do it. The same is true of electrocardiograms and basic X-rays of the chest and bones. Many homes have their own electrocardiogram machines and we also have a noninvasive bladder scan that allows us to measure the residual urine and workings of the bladder without an invasive and painful catheterization. This is a test that is easy to perform and I have yet to see a hospital use it at the bedside as we do.

On the more sophisticated side, we can order other tests such as sonograms (echo tests) of the abdomen to evaluate the liver, gallbladder, and pancreas. We can, within a few days, obtain a portable cardiac ultrasound to evaluate the pumping action of the heart and the competence of the heart valves. In questions about circulation, we can obtain Doppler studies of both the arteries and veins of the legs. Because the companies that provide these services have many competitors, they are happy to sit down and revise their services according to our needs. For example, the tests of arterial circulation were helpful but not adequate; they did not include the exact ratio of how the legs were receiving circulation. I met with the account manager who had heard similar things from other homes. Within a month, he had sent a tech for training in this other technique and now each arterial Doppler includes this ratio. I can't imagine many hospitals in my area being that responsive.

One common reason for hospitalization is telemetry, which is a device that allows constant monitoring of the heart rhythm. This is particularly helpful in patients with rapid or irregular heart rhythms. I just heard of a nearby nursing home that provides this service for a limited number of beds. They have a cardiologist who is available to review rhythms and in so doing can avoid unnecessary stays in the hospital. Make no mistake, many of these advances help give the homes an edge over their competitors and are great for marketing and the bottom line. To me, it's a win-win.

As we discussed in a prior chapter on consultants, doctors who can travel to a nursing home and perform an examination there often prevent hospitalizations. Perhaps all that is needed is an outpatient CT scan or an endoscopy of the GI tract. The consultant might even help by explaining to the family that there is nothing to be gained from hospitalizing a loved one.

An Old Dog Learns New Tricks

There are also exciting new services on the horizon. A group of wound specialists recently approached us to see if they could help in our facility. Traditionally, it has been very hard to get specialized care for a leg wound or pressure sore in a nursing home. In fact, it was even hard to find a specialist who would see residents without a trip to the hospital. Currently, companies that sell special beds and wound equipment provide a wound-care nurse who travels to the home and provides an informal consultation. I am uncomfortable with this arrangement for several reasons. First, the nurses often recommend products that the company sells or rents—no surprise there. Second, the nurse often performs the consultation informally and will not commit to anything in writing. We also are never in a position to know the nurse's credentials. Of course we can ask, and they may well be certified as a specialist, but it removes a level of supervision that I would rather not cede.

In contrast, the wound-care group that approached me does not represent any supply company, allowed me to credential its consultants, has thorough follow-up, and provides some education to our nurses. The other major advantage is that they perform a minor procedure called debridement at the bedside. I do perform this procedure myself on patients, but most physicians do not, and in an era of increased malpractice litigation in nursing homes, I can't blame them. Debridement involves cutting and scraping away dead tissue from a wound in order to help it heal. It is often done with a scalpel and local anesthesia and should be done as early as it is needed, otherwise the wound can fester and worsen quickly. Early attention to a wound is paramount in keeping that resident out of the hospital. It also protects the facility and physician from liability.

Make no mistake, this wound group is a company with an aggressive business plan. I wouldn't use the group for more minor wounds that I feel my staff and I can treat. But in homes where the doctors visit only once a month, the service cannot be beat. The group's success will depend on its supply of competent physicians or "physician extenders" if it goes that route. While the services cost Medicare and the other insurance companies in the short run, I do think that by doling out ounces of prevention, they will save pounds of costs down the road.

A Reality Check

There are several caveats to this antihospitalization trend. First, in more rural areas the availability of mobile lab and X-ray companies may be limited. Second, there will be a profusion of offers to facilities for treatments that may not be warranted or medically indicated. I will leave it up to the administrators and health economists to keep an eye on that score. Third, the readiness of specialists to set foot in nursing homes and effect change there is limited right now. I do think that will change as competition forces them to seek new venues in which to apply their art.

You may already have had the experience that when a frail elder ends up in an emergency room, there is a great sucking sound. Just the appearance of mental confusion, which may have been there for years, will sway the emergency room doctor to admit the person first and ask questions later. There is, of course, wide variability and—to no one's surprise—it depends on the availability of beds. Many states have done the hard work of cutting down on the number of hospital beds. The culture in those communities is to take care of people at the nursing homes; they will only be sent back from the ER anyway. In my area, this mostly happens in the dead of winter when influenza and ice accidents collude to fill the hospitals to capacity. Even so, many of the doctors in our area still don't get it and reflexively send the residents to the ER.

Can we talk about dignity and comfort? Because of overcrowding, many ERs are storehouses for patients waiting to go to a room. After I have seen someone in the ER and stabilized them, he or she can often wait a day or two to go upstairs to a real bed. This depends on the time of year, but sometimes the ER is even on "divert," which means it is full and the ambulance takes the resident to another hospital farther away. It makes visiting more of a stretch for the family and it means the care of the resident is assigned to a doctor who has never seen the resident before. Sitting on a hard gurney, lights at full blast and noises aplenty, it's no wonder that my residents become agitated. The agitation often prompts an order for a sedative that knocks the patient out and muddles the picture even more. In my experience, almost anyone with gray hair and a modicum of confusion from a nursing home is tied down (i.e., restrained). In short, it's a bleak scene and if you can do anything reasonable to prevent it, you'll be doing your loved one a true act of kindness.

Surprising Scenarios

I would like to provide some scenarios that can be addressed in the nursing home rather than in the hospital. Some may come as a surprise. Let me preface this by saying that aside from the medical aspects and details of care, quality-of-life issues often prevail. Let's say that you have a 102-year-old aunt, who has suffered from dementia for seven years and is now so incapacitated that she needs help in all her activities. She cannot feed herself and needs to be transported out of bed by two aides or nurses. She does not recognize you and can only say a few words. Or you can substitute your own example of someone maybe not quite as debilitated, but whom you know *would never want to be living like this*. Even if you don't wish to give up, the nursing home can provide very good care and even aggressive care without the tumult and dislocation that a transfer to the hospital entails. An acute illness *may* even be the time when you as a loved one are able to allow the person a peaceful passing. As I say to my patients and always apologize in advance for saying it: *No one lives forever*. If you believe in the Almighty, it may be God's way of taking someone home. If not, it's an opportunity to die with dignity and with comfort that, I would argue, can better be provided in a nursing home than in a hospital. There are groups like hospice that can try to ensure comfort within the nursing home. So always look at the big picture and don't let anyone sell you a bill of goods. There are many perverse incentives in the Medicare system that encourage hospitalizations. The doctors, nursing homes, and hospitals all stand to profit *and* perceive of it as a way to reduce their legal exposure. The choice is your loved one's and yours.

* * *

The quintessential case of someone "needing" hospitalization is a heart attack (myocardial infraction), right? I can tell you that I've taken care of many a heart attack at the nursing home. I can't give you survival statistics, but I've never had a family upbraid me for not transferring a resident. Most of my patients were more comfortable, less stressed, and less confused sticking it out in their own beds. If a patient is frail or has significant dementia, it is unlikely that any invasive procedures such as coronary angiographies and angioplasties will be performed. If they develop complications, such as congestive heart failure or low blood pressure, we can usually deal with it in the home. If not, we can always change course and transfer out at that point. Most of these complications are witnessed within the first day or two of a heart attack and tend not to be as common in the frail elderly. It is unusual for an elder in a nursing home to suffer "the big one," because of the way the heart responds to years of gradual narrowing of its main coronary arteries. I can only recall one "transmural" or major heart attack in a nursing home patient of mine in twenty years of practice. The others are what we call subendocardial—the body has protected itself by alternate pathways for blood and oxygen called collaterals. We can provide oxygen, aspirin, beta-blockers, and morphine, which are still the main ingredients on the heart attack menu in a hospital. Most of our residents have an order *not* to perform CPR in the event of a cardiac arrest (which *infrequently* is the outcome of a heart attack), and that would be the case in the hospital, too. As I discuss in chapter 12, the studies of CPR performed on the frail elderly show the success rate is abysmal, so your aunt would not be missing much anyway (except the broken ribs and needle sticks that are part of the CPR experience).

*   *   *

Infections are a common precipitant to hospitalization. Apply the quality-of-life rule as you would to any decision to transfer your loved one out of the home. Pneumonia and urinary tract infections can sometimes be mild, but can also be severe and life threatening. When life threatening, they cause a picture known as sepsis, marked by high fever, low blood pressure, mental confusion, possible dehydration, and damage to other organs, such as the heart, kidneys, or liver. In these situations, the key to survival is giving antibiotics quickly and fluid if it is needed. Many residents can get started at the nursing home on oral antibiotics and fluids by mouth and can turn the corner in their own bed. If the route of hospitalization is chosen, one must wait for the ambulance, an ER bed, and an evaluation by the ER doctor. It can be several hours before they initiate active treatment. In our home, the care can be started immediately. This is not the case in all homes, so you must have an appreciation for the level of care and monitoring in your reference home. Are the nurses at the home attentive and do the doctors have a real presence? If the home has a nurse practitioner or a physician's assistant, all the better as they can evaluate the resident quickly and initiate care. Sometimes the physicians know the patient well enough that they are confident in starting the treatment by telephone and then seeing the patient in a few days.

Some residents of nursing homes develop an internal blood clot in the leg vein known as a deep vein thrombosis or DVT. The leg and foot often swell and become painful. The danger of a DVT is that it can break off and travel to the lungs where it becomes known as a pulmonary embolus or PE. In the past, blood clots like these required hospitalization. The accepted treatment was an intra-

venous blood thinner called Heparin. Heparin was largely sup-
planted by a group of medications released in the mid-1990s called
"low molecular weight heparins" of which enoxaparin (Lovenox)
and dalteparin (Fragmin) are but two examples. These are injected
subcutaneously, much like insulin. The dose is calculated according to the size of the patient and most of the time does not require
twice-a-day blood tests that are the bane of the original Heparin
treatment. Multiple studies have established the safety of these
injections over Heparin. In younger patients with clots, doctors
mostly treat in an outpatient fashion. The injections last only for
a few days and then are followed by six months of an oral blood
thinner known as warfarin (Coumadin). There are a few exceptions to this rule. A large lung clot can compromise the breathing
and/or circulation. But in general, if a doctor recommends hospitalization, you might want to ask his or her justification and why
he or she prefers that to nursing home injections.

Another condition that in the past required hospital treatment
was the stroke/TIA syndrome. A TIA (also called a mini-stroke,
though it really isn't) represents a syndrome that begins as a stroke
but reverses itself completely within a set period of time (twenty-
four hours). In frail older people, aggressive clot busters such as
TPA (see discussion in chapter 6) are usually more dangerous
than helpful. The main determinant in whether to consider TPA is
whether a clot or a hemorrhage causes the stroke. A clot prevents
blood flow much like a coronary artery clot causes a heart attack.
Neurologists now refer to a stroke as a "brain attack" exactly for
this reason. High blood pressure and other factors can cause the
less common hemorrhagic stroke in which a blood vessel bursts
to cause bleeding. Since the treatments are different, one usually

wants to know the *type* of stroke, and a "simple" CT scan without contrast dye can differentiate. I will sometimes send a resident to the ER to get a quick CT scan and make sure other medical issues are stable. If the stroke or TIA is from a clot, I usually bring the resident back to the home and start a blood thinner like aspirin. If hemorrhagic, it depends on the severity of the situation.

There are strokes and there are *strokes*. Many strokes are ill defined and result in mild weakness, slurred speech, and/or visual changes. Others are massive and result in difficulty swallowing and deterioration of mental function. While the temptation is to hospitalize for the more major strokes, the care may be more appropriate at the nursing home. If the quick CT scan approach was undertaken, a neurologist may be able to consult in the ER. He or she may tell you that the prognosis is grave no matter what you do. Also, if the resident suffers from severe dementia or for quality-of-life reasons wants no aggressive treatment in the event of a stroke (some living wills stipulate this), then also consider sending the resident back to the home. Hospice may be an option in these cases. The ER in our hospital now staffs a social worker who helps families through these decisions and informs them of all their options. She has a tough job but does it well. She recently convinced the family of one of my sickest and frailest patients that hospice was at last appropriate. I had sat with them many times before with the same goal but was not able to persuade them. I guess they just needed more time and patience.

One of the toughest syndromes is severe peripheral vascular disease, which can result in gangrene. This condition is caused by poor circulation to the legs. Its cause is the same atherosclerosis that causes heart attacks and strokes by blocking major arteries that feed blood and oxygen to the tissues that need them. Occasionally the blockages are sudden and can be diagnosed with special X-rays called angiograms in the hospital. If the vascular surgeons can pinpoint the blockage they can try to clear it with balloons or clot busters. More often, they will attempt a bypass operation very much like a heart bypass with which you may be more familiar. It's less risky than a heart bypass because the surgeon does not need to stop the heart and use special machines to take the place of the heart during surgery. Whatever the options, the older and more frail the patient, the more risky these procedures are. Most circulation problems in nursing home patients occur due to multiple levels of blockage in multiple arteries and are not amenable to these procedures.

Circulation problems like this often result in nonhealing ulcers of the feet and/or legs. As long as some blood is getting through, they have a chance of healing, and a vascular surgeon or wound specialist may be of help to the primary-care team. The tougher scenario is when the circulation utterly fails and areas of the feet begin to turn blue or black. That signifies dying (necrotic) tissue and results in gangrene. Some gangrene is "dry," that is, the tissue turns black but remains dry and uninfected. "Wet" gangrene has a nastier look and usually involves redness, odor, and infection.

Regardless, both conditions can be painful and often require strong narcotic medications. The combination of poor circulation, dying tissue, narcotics, and possible infection conspire to worsen the overall health of the person. This may result in death in a matter of days or weeks and hospice is often an important part of the care plan. Hospice essentially seeks comfort over cure (see chapter 12). If adequate pain control gets lost in the shuffle, the hospice team is aggressive in requesting and obtaining better care. Just a few weeks ago, I lost a woman in her late nineties with exactly this scenario. She died about a month after the gangrene set in. Hospice was involved and she had a comfortable passing. You may ask, "Why wasn't amputation performed? Wouldn't that have relieved the pain and extended her life?" In Bertha's case, she had suffered enough. The last eight years of her life were filled with operations, strokes, hospitalizations, depression, creeping confusion…you name it. She had even been on hospice before but had somehow survived. Her supremely loving family was adamant that God had provided an escape hatch; her time had come. She had lived a full life—a life worth living—and seen the births of many grandchildren and great-grandchildren. No more tests, no more hospitalizations, no more torment.

There are other times when amputation *can* make sense. In contrast to Bertha, a woman just a few doors down named Essie was in her late eighties and developed similar gangrene of one leg. We tried as best we could but nothing helped. Her family asked for an amputation and, to my surprise, Essie agreed. She was quite aware and though she suffered mild confusion due to her condition and the narcotics we gave her, she convinced me that she understood the pros and cons of amputation. In contrast to Bertha, Essie still took great pleasure in life. She listened to the Metropolitan Opera broadcasts on Saturday afternoons. She was a member of our music appreciation group. She knew when her family was coming and going and was proud of her granddaughter's academic accomplishments in high school. She wanted to trace the complete trajectory of her life. She still saw herself on the upswing and was hungry for every day she had left. With the amputation, there was a reasonable chance to be out of pain and to enjoy life as she knew it. Now a few years later, I can say she made the right choice. At the time, I wasn't so sure, but I do learn from my patients and hope that those lessons inform my care of others.

All this is predicated on you as a family member being part of the plan and understanding the pros and cons, the risks and the benefits. If you desire longevity at all costs, then hospitalize at all costs, but involve your loved one and listen to him. Do not be motivated by guilt or the feeling that because you cherish your loved one, you want all care at any cost. If he can still make decisions, then more power to him and have him participate in all discussions unless he cedes that to you. If he cannot make decisions, then substitute your judgment for his, but always hear his imaginary voice telling you what would be important to him at this time of his life. For a reality check, when I spend the time and explain these issues carefully to my patients or to the families of my patients, they mostly choose to remain in their own home...the nursing home. They literally choose to *live* without the hospital.

Getting What You Want

If you do not wish for hospitalization, how do you ensure that your wishes and your parent's wishes are observed? You may be familiar with the abbreviation "DNR" for Do Not Resuscitate, but you may not know that many nursing homes have a "DNH" preference as well. The H-word here is "hospitalize," as in Do Not Hospitalize. This is usually in addition to a DNR and stipulates that you do not wish your parent to be sent to the hospital. You may prefer not to commit to a DNH. Why not just address the issue when your parent gets sick? Well, in the real world of nursing homes, stuff happens. Frail nursing home patients quickly get sick. The home will call the doctor first, who may give an order at three in the morning to send your parent to the hospital and ask questions later. The home may then call you after the fact; the ambulance is already in the driveway. It is very hard to put the brakes on this juggernaut.

Also, no matter how many phone numbers, beeper numbers, e-mail addresses, and cell phones you leave, the home sometimes just can't seem to get hold of you. The first call you get is from the ER and then the process develops a life of its own. The doctor will tell you the orders have already been given, the blood was drawn, just "give it a few days and let's see what turns up." You can refuse hospitalization after that but it's hard to do unless the doctor takes your point of view. If you feel that you don't want the hospitalization, please take pains to avoid it with a proper DNH. The hospice movement has used DNHs to great advantage in order to prevent a dying or terminal patient from being sent out in violation of the principles of palliative and comfort care.

What if the nursing home refuses a DNH request or says it has no such policy? You appeal to the medical director or director of social work but to no avail. In *my* view, that warrants a call to the state ombudsman as a denial of your loved one's rights as a resident to refuse care. I can't guarantee what the ombudsman will do, but it's worth a try and you might be able to effect changes at the home. Do *not* accept the status quo. As Gandhi said, "Be the change you wish to see in the world."

A DNH order does not mean that the home will keep your parent under any circumstance. Like a DNR, it can be rescinded at any time. It does assure (I would hope) that the home consults you before any decisions are made; the presumption is to keep your loved one in the nursing home, in her own bed. The few possible exceptions to this include traumatic injuries such as a skin tear that might need suturing in the ER and a fall with a hip fracture that might require surgery for relief of pain. If a resident is in the last throes of life and death seems imminent, a DNH would likely trump a hip fracture. Short of that, though, hip surgery usually relieves pain more efficiently and the fracture might trump the DNH.

Medicare and the Search for Alternatives

Medicare regards the frequent hospitalization of nursing home residents as a marker for poor care. Medicare keeps records by state and the variation is remarkable. For example, in 2002, for a five-month stretch, almost 25% of nursing home residents in New Jersey were hospitalized, while in Idaho the figure was a mere 5%. Medicare's interest is partly financial and partly quality of care. Discrepancies like this, though, are so glaring that it puts fire in the belly of the beast.

In the mid-1980s, Medicare began looking for demonstration projects to address this issue. The most successful of these was a program created by two nurse practitioners in 1987 called Evercare. It is now operational in forty states and has thousands and thousands of members. It is part of Ovations, a division of UnitedHealth Group. For full disclosure, our nursing home joined the program in 2006 and it so impressed me that I began working on a part-time basis for Evercare later that year. Though I am employed by Evercare, my views do not necessarily reflect those of UnitedHealth Group.

By rearranging the insurance and clinical ends of care, Evercare seeks to reduce the rate of hospitalization. In a nutshell, Evercare stresses preventive care and discerning changes of condition early to avert the possibility that a frail elder "needs" to be hospitalized. Gratis to the nursing home, Evercare places skilled nurse practitioners that work in partnership with the doctors and nurses of the home to supplement the care. The home and the resident derive the benefits of the extra care for free. Evercare also has permission from Medicare to reverse some of the traditional financial incentives to hospitalize. It pays doctors more for seeing residents early and often *at* the nursing home.

Evercare also waives the so-called three-day rule, which under regular Medicare pays the nursing home much higher rates for *sub-acute* care upon return if the patient has stayed for at least three days. The three-day rule practically encourages homes to send residents to the hospital. Under Evercare, nursing homes can now receive higher payment for skilled days while treating "in place" *without* sending residents to the hospital. The experience across the country is that these changes reduce hospitalizations by about 40% *and* people actually survive a bit longer! Evercare helps Medicare save money and improve care. The nursing home makes more money or remains whole while improving care, and the residents and families, as surveys show, love the extra TLC and insurance benefits that are part of the Evercare package.

I present this not as free advertising for Evercare—I have already disclosed my position—but to tell you how a bright idea by two people who cared about care translated into a structure that promotes what geriatricians espouse. A potential stumbling block for Evercare is that the program depends on the availability of well-trained and compassionate nurse practitioners; they may be in short supply in the future. Evercare is taking great pains as a company to build a pipeline that will ensure its supply. You might want to ask the nursing home if it has a partnership with Evercare, and if so, ask to meet the nurse practitioner assigned to the home. Know that enrollment is voluntary and can be reversed on a monthly basis.

If You Still Don't Believe Me...

In closing this very important chapter, I recall a few vignettes shared with me by friends. One of these friends had a mom who was hospitalized just before she died in a very frail and debilitated state. I had taken care of her years ago when I did more outpatient work and she happened to be a favorite of mine. She was a lovely human being with a heart of unalloyed gold. She suffered from a congenital condition called alkaptonuria, a disease that turned her urine black and crippled her joints with arthritis. She used to relate to me stories of growing up in the early part of the last century with a problem with which few people were familiar. There were no support groups or chat rooms and she made her own way through an unusual life. In the hospital, my friend went to visit her and noted her mother was in pain. After some time, the sheets and covers were taken down and it was discovered that a tourniquet had been left on her arm after a blood draw. The arm was near circulatory collapse and had turned color. Is hospital care better care?

The other story was from a colleague who is a nurse. She had become close to a family whose mom had been talked into being hospitalized for trouble breathing. She ended up being placed on a ventilator with a breathing tube down her throat into her windpipe. Because the doctors had described it as their last chance (doctors often phrase it as doing "everything"), the family agreed to it, saying they were made to feel they "didn't have a choice."

For those of you who have not witnessed someone in this condition on a ventilator, it is one of the most difficult of scenes. The breathing tube is a constant irritation—often terrifying and painful. It comes as part and parcel of the whole ICU scene with different tubes, alarms, needles, doctors, nurses, and little chance to sleep. The patient generally needs to be sedated and given morphine, but these have to be reduced in order to wean the person from the breathing machine. If the weaning can't be done, the doctors within a week to ten days may convince the family to perform a tracheostomy, which is the opening of a hole through the neck into the windpipe.

Needless to say, ventilators save thousands of lives each year and are a standard part of general anesthesia. In a weak and fragile nursing home resident that more than likely will die within a few weeks to months after being on a ventilator, it can also be seen as cruel and unusual. The mother survived and in a weak voice upon returning to the nursing home told her daughter, "Don't ever do that to me again." Only weeks later, the mom developed the same problems and the daughter this time made her a DNH and let her mother go quietly and comfortably in accord with her own wishes. Whatever do-good instincts or guilt that induces a child to do "everything" for her mom can be more than offset by the look of pain and anguish on your loved one's face that will be etched into your memory for years to come. No choice? You *always* have a choice.

10

Falls and Restraints

Until recently, restraints were seen as the solution to falls in elderly nursing home residents. Any discussion of one involved the other. Falls are extremely common in the community and epidemic in long-term care. At least half of elderly nursing home residents experience a fall each year and the percentage would be even higher if so many were not bed bound. Some falls indicate that a medical issue or a subtle stroke has occurred, while some are "multifactorial" and harder to diagnose and prevent. Good homes study individual falls, fall rates, locations of the falls, timing of the falls, etc. They seek to understand how to take a micro and macro approach to minimize the chance of a fall in the future.

A Primer on Falls

We doctors say that falls can be caused by either extrinsic or intrinsic causes (which is another way of saying external or internal causes). Most often, a combination of the two is responsible. The most prevalent extrinsic causes have to do with the physical environment. Perhaps the furniture is in an awkward spot or there's just too much of it. Taking a trip to the bathroom at two A.M. and navigating between the straits of a reclining chair, a tray table, and a lamp can cause a moment's unsteadiness and a fall. A younger person's balance, vision, and reflexes are sharp enough that the ship can be righted. An older person does not have the same ability and being just a bit off-kilter will surely result in a fall.

A woman named Bernice used to live at our nursing home. Bernice walked without a cane or walker but had a wide-based gait that indicated a subtle balance problem. She also had mild Alzheimer's disease, which impaired her judgment and ability to process spatial cues. She began falling and was lucky not to have injured herself. We scoured her room and found that someone had moved her telephone to a high table. Her very alert nurse's aide watched Bernice pick up the phone and noted that when she did so, she lifted her arm and twisted her neck in such a way that she developed a moment's vertigo and began listing to one side. The aide grabbed her and reported it to us. Arthritis of the neck can affect older people in such a way that mechanoreceptors—little gyroscopes for the body—are thrown off and cause dizziness. We moved the phone to a lower and better location, and the falls ceased.

Deciphering what causes falls is sleuth work. Someone on the team has to take the time and the initiative to case the joint and pick up the scent of the trail. Many times, this is the nurse or nurse's aide, which was the case with Bernice. Other times, the family is the one spending the most time with the resident and should feel free to chime in with any information. Try to see if the falls are happening at a particular time or in a certain place. Sometimes the resident is slipping on urine in the room or in the bathroom. The staff should take the resident on a fixed schedule every two hours to avoid incontinence or leakage. Sometimes the falls occur in a hallway just after the floor has been washed. Because of a visual problem and/or dementia, the resident does not comprehend what the posted WET FLOOR warning signs mean. The staff can keep the resident busy during this brief period and avoid an accident waiting to happen. Or perhaps the housekeepers are not even *using* the warning placards as they should. Is it possible for the housekeepers to alter their schedule so that they avoid mopping during busy transit times?

The nurse's care plan must describe what assistive devices the resident needs to be able to get up out of bed each day. Many residents use a walker or cane, or cruise around in a wheelchair. If these devices are not juxtaposed to the bed, the resident will need to go searching or may not remember to look at all. This leaves them unsafe and vulnerable. The care plan should read like an interior designer's book and list what should be where in the room. Would a commode (i.e., a potty) next to the bed help avert the two A.M. sojourn to the bathroom? Does the resident need one bed rail up to grab on to in order to get out of bed? Without the bed rail, she may slip to the side of the bed in an awkward lunge and tumble to the floor. By the same token, are two bed rails up when your parent doesn't need them, but they force her to crawl to the end of the bed and fall in doing so? Are the shoes too loose or is your mother vain enough to still be wearing hazardous high heels? So play detective, join the "force," and solve the puzzle.

Intrinsic (or internal) causes of falls are legion. Whereas with extrinsic causes, anyone can offer an opinion, decoding the intrinsic causes may require a nursing or medical degree. The first item of business is to be sure that your parent is really falling and not fainting or having seizures. The latter is less common and usually

someone witnesses shaking movements or severe fatigue and confusion following a seizure. Fainting (syncope) can be very hard to
detect. It is most common in people with heart or blood pressure
problems. The common pathway leading to a faint is a drop in
blood pressure to the point where the blood and its nutrients do
not reach the brain. The body's protective response is to assume
a horizontal position so that the blood can reach the brain more
easily and not need to overcome gravity. When the brain receives
blood again, it quickly revives and within ten to fifteen minutes
can be reasonably back to business as usual.

How low does the blood pressure need to drop before syncope
occurs? That really depends on the person, but in general, once the
top number (systolic blood pressure) falls below ninety, an older
person is likely to feel woozy and begin to faint. Unfortunately,
if the person falls and is on the ground for several minutes, by the
time the nurse gets the person back to bed, the blood pressure may
return to normal and no one will suspect a faint as opposed to
an ordinary fall. The trick is to have a level of suspicion aroused
by the pattern and timing of the falls. It is helpful for the doctor
to check the blood pressure in both a lying and standing position
(postural signs). If the pressure drops by 15–20% or more, this can
suggest a fainting disorder.

Factors that predispose someone to syncope or fainting are
probably too numerous to list and many of the causes conspire
with other causes. In the nursing home resident, dehydration is a
common basis and this can be accentuated by medications that
lower the blood pressure. As people age, their blood pressure tends
to rise, but this is not always the case; some people are on too
many blood pressure medications and live at a pressure that just
barely keeps them conscious. If a new medication is added or they
become dehydrated due to hot weather, it can literally tip them

over to a faint. Diuretic medications (water pills) can be useful for treating congestive heart failure, but as conditions change, the resident may not need the same dosage. Maintaining too high a dose can cause dehydration and syncope.

As we talked about chapter 6 on medications, Dr. Lewis Lipsitz characterized a syndrome related to lowering of the blood pressure after a meal called post-prandial hypotension. This compounds with the effects of medications and dehydration.

Internal bleeding can cause so much loss of blood and fluid that the body has little left with which to generate a blood pressure; it can result in fainting. Sometimes this is obvious with visible blood in the stool or black tarry-looking stools. The blood pressure may be low and the blood count may reveal anemia. Sometimes, as happened to a patient of mine some years back, it is subtler. The patient was a man we called "The Captain" because he always wore a captain's hat and a blue blazer; he also spent a lot of time sunning himself on the patio of the home. He was a dead ringer for Tony Curtis in his male role in *Some Like It Hot*. The Captain, who *had* been quite steady on his feet, began falling and we attributed this to his progressive dementia. Because he was tanned, we missed the fact that he was profoundly anemic from internal bleeding. We found him several days after a fall in a pool of bloody stool in his bed. His blood pressure was very low and he was barely conscious. The falls had more than likely been individual faints. At that time, I did not carry with me the small bottle of special fluid and stool-testing cards that can detect hidden or "occult" blood in the stool. If I had it with me and had thought enough to test the stool, I might have made a difference and avoided his transfer to the hospital. He had a large bleeding ulcer, but survived after receiving several pints of blood. I do carry those cards and fluids with me now and salute The Captain every time I use them.

There are also underlying heart problems that can cause syncope. The main valve of the heart, the aortic valve, can become too tight (stenotic) and not allow blood reliably to get to the brain. This usually causes a fairly loud heart murmur and other symptoms, such as chest pain and shortness of breath. An echocardiogram (also known as an echo or a cardiac ultrasound) can reveal this as well. Abnormal heart rhythms can also result in syncope from either too rapid a heartbeat or, more commonly, too slow a heartbeat. If an examination and plain electrocardiogram (EKG) do not disclose this easily, the doctor may need to order a twenty-four-hour Holter monitor. This is a portable cardiogram that the person wears strapped to his body that records every heartbeat in a day. Patients with dementia will often remove or disconnect the mildly annoying apparatus.

Once fainting has been excluded, other intrinsic factors should come to mind. Are there any neurological findings that are apparent or does the resident suffer from a neurological disease that affects the gait? Parkinson's disease classically affects balance and gait and causes falls. We can aggressively treat Parkinson's with a new arsenal of drugs. Unfortunately, the older one is, the less likely it is *pure* Parkinson's and the more likely there will be side effects from the medications. Alzheimer's disease, as it enters its later stages, results in perception, balance, gait, and/or behavioral issues that can cause falling. Strokes or, for that matter, any medical condition that weakens the body can cause a fall. Pneumonia is a condition that in younger people produces fever, cough, and blood-tinged sputum. In the elderly, these symptoms may be absent. In their place come confusion, lethargy, and sometimes falls. Similar results can accrue from a heart attack, a urinary infection, or a stroke. These are known as sentinel falls.

There are yet more ways that a frail elder can fall. I saw two

patients just this past year who were brought to me after falling. They each said they could not walk, but when we obtained
a careful history, it turned out the change was caused by pain in
the ankle joint. Examination revealed hot, red, exquisitely painful
joints. Blood work revealed elevated uric acid levels that indicate
gout. Even without the blood tests, the gout was fairly obvious and
at least merited a treatment course. Some treat gout with nonsteroidal anti-inflammatories like ibuprofen (Motrin, Advil) or cele-
coxib (Celebrex). In the elderly, I prefer an older medicine called
colchicine, which is a *specific* treatment for gout. If colchicine
eradicates the pain, then you've got yourself a diagnosis. We used
colchicine and had those ankle joints feeling better and those folks
walking safely again in a matter of days.

There are many more mundane reasons that an older person
with joint disease can fall. The most common of these is plain old
arthritis (known as osteoarthritis or degenerative joint disease).
Arthritis affects the knee and hip joints more than any other joints.
Without treatment, and often despite treatment, standing and
walking become painful. This starts a vicious cycle of the person
walking less to avoid the pain, the muscles beginning to atrophy
due to disuse, the gait becoming less steady due to muscle atrophy,
and the person eventually falling.

Severe arthritis can even destabilize the joint itself and cause
the joint to buckle. A failed joint can precipitate a fall. X-rays, history, and examination can usually nail down a diagnosis. Treatment almost always involves analgesics to lessen the pain along
with some type of physical therapy. The therapist may use other
modalities, such as heat or ice or a brace, to help the joint and prescribe a cane or walker to reduce the strain on the joint.

If a joint has failed completely, usually indicated by pain even
at night while resting, a joint replacement may be contemplated.

While these operations can help walking, they are no walk in the park. The surgery can be risky and the therapy needed afterward is intense, especially for knee replacements; in frail nursing home patients, replacement is rarely an option. Orthopedists are researching other less invasive ways to remold a joint, so keep your ears to the ground. Other forms of arthritis, such as rheumatoid arthritis, are less common but can also weaken joints.

Sometimes a fall or other trauma can result in a crack in the hip joint that over time evolves into a fracture. The original trauma may not have been reported or seemed minor and no X-rays were taken. If such a resident falls a second time, and complains of any pain from the pelvis, hip, or knee, an X-ray may document an occult fracture. Hip pain can sometimes show up as knee pain—a phenomenon we call "referred" pain.

What if the team makes an exhaustive evaluation and nothing treatable turns up? Falls of this kind almost always merit a course of physical therapy and a thorough review of the environmental situation. Maybe the person's room is too far from the dining area and she runs out of gas by the time she reaches it. If this is the cause of a fall, perhaps the resident can move to a closer room. Perhaps she needs to be reminded to use a walker or have a nurse's aide be sure to walk *with* her to each meal. This needs to be memorialized as part of the written care plan. The team often misses these little things and plunks someone into a wheelchair. The problem with a wheelchair is that the resident walks very little, the muscles weaken by the day, and walking becomes even more hazardous.

Wheelchairs certainly save staff time, make mealtime more efficient, and are sometimes necessary. Often the staff and you can reach a compromise whereby your parent walks on the nursing unit but uses the wheelchair to go off the unit for an event in another part of the home. If your parent is forced to use it, the physical therapist must be involved in ordering the correct chair. It should fit the body shape and be cleaned often. Residents in our home have a nasty habit of saving fruit, milk, and rolls in the recesses of their wheelchairs and they can become mobile trash dumps.

Some residents can actually propel themselves with their feet as if they were still walking. This is preferable since they maintain some independence and keep their legs strong. Others need the footrests and someone to push them.

If a resident has a weak arm from a stroke or arthritis, she may need a special axle on the wheelchair that allows for one-armed use. Without it, she will literally go in circles. If she is too weak to propel herself but still wishes independence, an occasional resident will be able to negotiate an electric wheelchair The chairs are very expensive and insurance companies, not to mention Medicare, are tough about reimbursement. The staff must be very careful that the residents can use them safely without morphing them into bumper cars.

I cared for a lovely woman who had had a stroke and was left after months of therapy still unable to use a standard wheelchair. She initially handled a powered chair well but developed other medical problems that made her unsafe. She not only banged herself up many a time but began running into and hurting other residents. She was aware enough to know that this was her last independent link to the world and was furious when we took it away from her. We gave her every chance to regain its use and even originated a kind of "driver's ed" course, but all to no avail.

If the resident falls and we don't wish to curtail her walking or she and the family refuse to curtail the walking, then we enter a kind of "prevent defense." We understand that the resident is at high risk for injury, but restraining her in any way will lead to greater weakness and, in an anxious or demented person, may cause agitation and paranoia. We then utilize several maneuvers to maximize safety. The simplest and cheapest of these is the hip protector mentioned briefly in chapter 7. These work well and have been successful in the nursing homes, less so in community studies. The problem with them is they are worn like hockey pads and many residents, especially those with dementia, remove them. Nevertheless, hip protectors are underutilized and if your parent falls, you should request them.

If the fall happens from bed and bed rails don't do the trick, the staff should consider either a bed alarm or a low bed. Bed rails are two-edged swords and while they can help prevent falls, many residents simply climb out over them and the result is a more dangerous fall from a higher position. Bed alarms are pressure-sensitive strips that the staff places under the sheets. When a person at risk for falls begins to get out of bed, the alarm triggers and sends out a piercing sound to the staff. This sounds great in theory but usually only alerts the staff to a fall that has already taken place. The chance of an alarm notifying the staff soon enough to quickly get in the room to prevent a fall is slim to none. In addition, alarms often misfire. This inures the staff to the sound and precisely defeats their purpose. The sound is horrifyingly loud and ruins the quiet on a nursing home unit. Bed alarms have become the car alarms of nursing homes and can awaken an entire neighborhood of residents. No wonder I'm asked for so many sleeping pills! Rumor has it that state and federal surveyors are contemplating banning bed alarms altogether. This would have to come from the government as homes now see the lack of an alarm for a falling resident as negligence and exposure to a lawsuit.

Alarms come in another flavor and that is an alarm for a chair or wheelchair. These work a bit better in that the person is usually in a common area for a meal or activity, not tucked away in her room, and staff is present to act on the alarm.

Even so, sometimes the chair alarms outlive their usefulness. I recently witnessed a woman who had been admitted to us several weeks before in a frail and deconditioned state. She had several medical problems that had been treated successfully and was a frequent faller. Despite her dementia, she did nicely in physical therapy and made great progress. The staff used a chair alarm that in the beginning did not go off very much. The night I happened to be on the unit, I saw her get up out of her chair and make a quick and steady lap around the dining area. She was so fast that the staff could barely keep up with her. Each time, the alarm blared and disturbed the peace of the unit. And each time, the staff placed her back in the chair with a warning about her risk of falling. This must have happened ten times in fifteen minutes when I finally asked the nurses to remove the alarm. Our therapy had actually *worked*. What was the point of it if not to have her walk by herself and so get rid of the alarm? I have seen a few alarms that instead of sounding like an air-raid siren have a soothing voice reminding the resident to sit down. I don't know how well they work, but my eardrums appreciate the effort.

When all else fails, and the resident continues to fall out of bed, we opt sometimes for a low bed. This means different things in different homes. The goal is that since the fall will happen, make the fall as safe as it can be. The bed is literally lowered toward the floor so that the resident falls onto a mat or mattress. Occasionally we have the bed only a foot off the floor. Once we even had the resident sleeping on a mattress *on* the floor. Most commonly, if the bed is an electric bed, we have it in its lowest position when the resident is in bed. The toughest thing about a low bed is that the staff has to get down on their hands and knees to perform care on the resident and to clean and make the bed. This can be back-breaking so the electric bed is a nice convenience. It can be raised when the staff needs to care for the resident. The electric beds are expensive and many homes cannot afford them so they must take a case-by-case approach. To place all residents in low beds would be impractical and irresponsible. Not to use them at all, equally so. A good physical therapist and/or nursing staff should be familiar with other devices that can prevent falls. There are special reclining chairs from which it is hard to get up by oneself. There are concave mattresses whose shape prevents a resident from climbing out of it. Unfortunately, these limit the residents' ability to move and can be classified as restraints.

The Untie the Elderly campaign began to gather steam in the late 1980s following the OBRA regulations. The Moses figure of this movement was a social worker named Carter Catlett Williams. I remember being present at one of the first hearings in Washington, D.C., that addressed the rampant use of restraints in nursing homes. Ms. Williams, with her regal bearing and flowing mane of white hair, was a most compelling speaker. Her thesis was not so much that restraints can be frankly dangerous (which they can be), but that tying up our elders was blatantly inhuman. It also didn't hurt her cause that she was married to Dr. T. Franklin Williams, who was the director of the National Institute on Aging. Her work, seen now almost twenty years later, has resulted in the lowest restraint use ever in U.S. nursing homes. Interestingly, these changes have barely taken hold in acute care hospitals. In this respect as with many geriatric concerns, the nursing homes are light-years ahead of our acute care partners.

What exactly is a restraint? A formal definition from Medicare is: "A restraint is any manual method or physical or mechanical device, material, or equipment that immobilizes or reduces the ability of a patient to freely move his arms, legs, body, or head." In some definitions, bed rails are considered restraints, though in practice, surveyors generally give a pass on bed rails. Medications that seek to sedate are technically considered chemical restraints, but surveyors tend to regard them under the "unnecessary medication" rules. Chest/vest restraints and wrist restraints, are the two most common types of restraints found in hospitals. You will be hard-pressed to find a nursing home that even stocks these items, let alone applies them.

A chest restraint is worn like a sweater or a vest and tethers the patient by his torso to the bed. It is ubiquitous in acute care hospitals. Several years ago, I saw some disturbing ads from the Posey Company (so major a producer of these that the vest restraints are known simply as "Poseys"), which feature young, smiling, carefree, buxom models wearing these restraints.

Wrist restraints go around the wrists and tie the patient to the bed frame, severely restricting his or her movements. They are used either to keep someone in bed that may otherwise get up, wander, and/or fall, or to prevent a patient from pulling out an IV line or catheter. One might ask, in a totally subversive way, if the patient demonstrates such resistance to care, is it not a sign that he or she really does not wish to be treated in that way and in that setting? The retort is usually that the patient is so demented, she doesn't know *what* she wants. In my book, if she is so unable to be a part of her own care, then what exactly are we accomplishing? In a more practical vein, the restraints cause severe agitation, which begets more sedatives, which begets immobility, which begets bedsores and pneumonia.

There are also reported cases of asphyxiation from vest restraints slipping up around a patient's throat and cutting off air. Families are often horrified that their loved one, who may have existed in the nursing home for years without a restraint, has them slapped on as soon as he or she hits the ER. They need to know that if they wish their loved one to be hospitalized, they are at the mercy of a culture very different from the nursing home. You are not in Kansas anymore! Don't get me wrong, hospitals are not gulags, and their needs and goals are different from ours in long-term care. Most recently, Medicare has cited a number of acute care hospitals for poor care with regard to restraints, so look for positive changes soon.

In nursing homes, the rules for restraints are reasonably clear. They may be used once all other reasonable alternatives have failed. According to state and federal regulations, the staff must foster the "highest practicable" level of independence. If you have tried alternatives and a risk/benefit analysis shows restraints to be less risky than not using them, you must use the least restrictive ones. There should be a note in the chart or a flow sheet from the nursing staff showing the rationale for applying the restraint and documenting what else has failed. There must be a doctor's order for the restraint and a medical diagnosis must justify the order.

For example, a resident is at risk for falls due to severe dementia. The dementia has come to such a pass that the ability to judge what a chair is and how to sit down are lost. The resident falls to the ground every time he attempts to sit down. The team has tried different approaches that have all failed and is honestly concerned that the resident will break a hip. Physical therapy has failed. An order from the doctor reads, "Seat belt in wheelchair to prevent falls. Diagnosis is Alzheimer's disease with poor judgment and safety awareness." In our home, we call the family and document that they understand and agree. The restraint should, according to regulation, be released on a fixed schedule every day. There also must be scheduled periodic reviews to determine if the restraint is still necessary. Do all homes follow these rules? Certainly not, but most come close. The use of restraints is dramatically lower than it had been and Medicare actually reports the percentage of residents in restraints as part of its report card on nursing homes. There are even restraint-free homes now, which used to be unthinkable. Chalk one up for culture change. Ms. Williams, along with other pioneers like Dr. Bill Thomas of the Eden Alternative, have brought about a sea change in how we care for our residents.

While our home is not restraint-free, we have lowered our use of restraints significantly. The only devices we use are the seat belts mentioned above and a cushion called, affectionately, a "lap buddy." When we first use a seat belt, we try one with a clasp buckle in the front that the resident can release by herself. If she demonstrates that she can release it, then it is not a restraint and serves more as a reminder not to get up without help. If the resident cannot release it, then we *do* register it as a restraint. The lap buddy is a cross between a cushion and a lap tray. It looks like a comfortable vinyl cushion that is notched and fits between the patient's lap and the arms of the wheelchair. It has the effect of preventing the resident from rising unattended but allows some wiggle room. Of course, some residents are strong and can pry it loose. We even had one resident who used it as a weapon and rolled around the halls hitting others in wheelchair polo. Needless to say, we took it away as the risks outweighed the benefits. If these devices are used to position properly the resident who might otherwise slip down out of the wheelchair, then it may not be a restraint.

Physicians may use restraints on an emergency basis. If the resident is in danger of causing *imminent* harm to herself or someone else, then the physician may call in a twenty-four-hour emergency order. The team must review the appropriateness of this every twenty-four hours and eventually go through the usual algorithm for long-term restraint use. Emergency restraint protocols are meant to cover weekends and nights. Many of these residents are precarious enough to need another setting within the home or another venue outside the home.

What if your loved one is falling or has fallen in the past? You've requested that the home uses a restraint, but it objected. You attend a family meeting where your request is discussed and the team explains that either the risks outweigh the benefits, or they have not tried enough other measures first. You insist that they must do what you say. It would be great to reach a compromise, but you *cannot* require the home to apply a restraint. If you feel that they have been through all feasible alternatives and your parent is in real danger, you might call the ombudsman's office and see what it says. It's rare and a bit more complicated if your loved one is alert and able to make her decisions. She probably has the right to a restraint if she feels it will improve her comfort or position or safety. In those cases, the team will most likely agree anyway and render it a moot point. It may seem intuitive that as we reduce restraints, the number of falls rises. Absolutely correct, but studies have shown that the serious injury rate stayed the same or decreased.

Falls will long be a regrettable concomitant of aging. Much like global warming, until we find a cure there will be stormy weather. As an industry, though, we have not rolled over and accepted restraints as part of our landscape. Quite the opposite: We have, in twenty years, unleashed a campaign to police them almost out of existence. Don't assume as a consumer that restraints are always advantageous. They can harm and they can even kill. The days

of doing what we want for our convenience and the days of families being able to demand what they want for peace of mind are
long gone. So raise a glass and toast Carter Williams of Untie the
Elderly fame. She proclaimed, "Let my people go," and countless
bonds have been loosed. She serves as a paradigm for fearless do-
gooders with a vision.

11

Bugs and Super-Bugs: Infections in Long-Term Care

Your eight-year-old has a runny nose and a fever, but you both want to visit Grandpa at the nursing home. Or, Grandpa has shingles and you want to bring your eight-year-old in for a visit. What is the right thing to do? Is plain old pneumonia contagious? Your mom just developed a positive skin test to TB. Is treatment necessary and is she contagious? This chapter provides the answers to these questions and more. It also talks about general precautions nursing homes should take to prevent the spread of infections.

Viruses and Influenza

While super-bugs are getting plenty of press right now, let's first talk about the plain vanilla bugs. Due to the rapidity with which they spread, viruses are nasty problems in nursing homes. The most common of these are the rhinoviruses that cause the common cold. A recurrent theme of this chapter will be that infections in the frail elderly are always more trouble than in the young; my residents start out in a weakened state with far less reserve. If you or I experience nasal congestion, a cough, and a low-grade fever when we catch a cold, my ninety-five-year-old with underlying emphysema may end up wheezing with pronounced shortness of breath. If the resident has heart disease as well (and upwards of 80% of ninety-five-year-olds do), the relative lack of oxygen may trigger angina or a heart attack. To complicate matters, there are many kinds of rhinoviruses and some are far more virulent than others, so it really depends on the season, the virus, and the state of your loved one.

The most feared virus, in a sense, is the influenza virus that comes in two types—type A and type B. Moreover, each year the particular kinds or subtypes of these viruses vary depending on where they originate in the world and how the genes of these viruses have changed or mutated. Most influenza viruses begin in Asia and over the course of a year wend their way to North America. Our influenza season begins in late October and usually lasts until March, though it can be a year-round phenomenon. The job of the vaccine makers is to guess about a year or two ahead of time which viruses will be upon us and against which they should make their vaccines. This is not a perfect science. More important, the older and frailer have weakened immune systems. The weaker the immune system, the less effective is the vaccine. That's the double whammy. The fragile immune system makes one more susceptible to the virus in the first place *and* lowers the chance that a vaccine will be effective. Vaccines depend on the body's immune system to generate antibodies against parts of the virus in the vaccine. Nevertheless, a recent study and editorial in the *New England Journal of Medicine* strongly supported influenza vaccination in elderly populations. Even after receiving the vaccine, though, one can catch the flu.

Because it lasts only about three months, the influenza vaccine should be given in late fall. In our home we usually vaccinate in early November. Researchers are now studying whether it makes sense to give a second dose in February or whether a much higher first-time dose will be more effective. The only viable reason *not* to receive the vaccine is an allergy to eggs (the vaccines are cultured on eggs). The vaccine will *not* give you influenza, though some still believe this.

The nursing home staff should receive the vaccine as well. If it does not and a worker happens to bring it into the facility, the flu will quickly overwhelm the ability of the vaccine to provide protection. While we strongly encourage it, we cannot mandate it and it is up to the good offices of our nursing leadership to see that it gets done. I am sad to say that in many facilities, the effort is lacking. While we're at it, what about family and visitors? They also should be vaccinated. We hold a family health fair once a year in the fall. It's a time when we offer free blood pressure checks, hearing exams, and the like. These are merely ways to get the families in the front door to offer to vaccinate them.

Most people can also receive the vaccine from their family doctor, county health office, or even at their drugstore. Short of the vaccine and because we cannot count on complete cooperation, we must advise families that if they are sick, please stay away! This is easier said than done and especially families with young children should take note. Kids are notorious carriers of viruses and should be encouraged to stay home even if they only have the sniffles. Please don't call me Scrooge, but I have seen the misery that a viral outbreak can wreak on a nursing home. It's no fun for the residents or the staff. Influenza can be deadly and tens of thousands of people each year die from it. Influenza can cause rapid dehydration, mental changes, painful muscle aches, and pneumonia, and spreads like wildfire.

The virus spreads through what we call "droplets." When one sneezes or coughs, little droplets of moisture carry the virus and spread it into the air infecting others that inhale the germs. If you must visit when you are sick, please ask the staff for a mask to wear; it will provide some protection to others. We sometimes place masks on our sick residents if we need to take them out of their room, but they are hard to keep in place. On that score, nursing homes should confine residents to their rooms if they are coughing or sneezing due to a virus. "Droplet precautions" are appropriate and mandate keeping the residents in their rooms as much as possible, bringing meals into their rooms, and having the staff wear masks and protective gowns. I sometimes see a resident with a respiratory virus sitting at a table of three other residents; it is a matter of a day or two until the others join in the cacophony of coughing. If you see this, point it out to the staff. If they refuse to remove the sick resident, then take your loved one immediately to her room and tell them I told you to do it!

Be obsessive about washing your hands. Most homes now carry hand sanitizers, which are alcohol-based gels and foams that work wonders (as shown by numerous studies). Use them liberally. You may notice that some nursing homes do not post notices outside residents' rooms when they are on "droplet precautions" or any other types of precautions. This is a sore point for me. Most acute care hospitals use the notices so that staff and visitors entering the room know how to act and what protective gear to wear. I took this issue to our state department of health and begged them to allow the notices on the doors in our home. The officials with whom I spoke fell back on the privacy issue and insisted that such posters compromised patient confidentiality. I have no idea why this is permitted in hospitals but not in nursing homes, but our compromise was to place a note on the door advising anyone who entered the room to see the nursing staff for further instruction.

What if your parent falls victim to influenza with a harsh cough, high fevers, muscle aches, and a positive nasal swab culture? You have most likely heard about medications that treat the flu. The good news is that these medications not only partially treat the flu but also can prevent it in the majority of people who receive it early enough. There were earlier versions of these medications called amantadine (Symmetrel) and rimantadine (Flumadine). They should not be used due to widespread resistance of Influenza A. (They are also not active against type B and can cause side effects.) That leaves two newer medications. One is named zanamivir (Relenza), which is taken in the form of inhaled powder and, as such, is difficult for nursing home residents to take effectively. It also can cause bronchospasm, which someone with influenza needs like a hole in the head. The other more common choice is oseltamivir (Tamiflu), which studies have shown is effective. When given to a resident who has the flu, it can shorten the severity of symptoms by a day or two. No great shakes, I guess, unless you have the flu; one less day of severe muscle aches and fever might be welcome indeed. To my mind, the major advantage of Tamiflu is that it is an effective prophylactic in those exposed to the flu. If a nursing unit develops a cluster—i.e., three or more cases—Tamiflu should be given to all the residents on the unit and the unit should be "closed." (It's preferable if influenza can be confirmed by at least one positive nasal or throat swab, but in practice this does not often happen.)

Let's take the closure first. This means mostly what it sounds like. No one on the unit, infected or not, should be allowed to leave the unit except for an emergency. There may need to be *some* give-and-take. An unaffected resident with a dental abscess needs to go to the dentist regardless, but by and large the home should maintain the closure until two full days pass without a new case of the flu. In most states, the home is also not supposed to admit new patients to a unit that is closed. (We try not to use the antiquated word *quarantined*.) This is the tough part, because new residents are the lifeblood of a facility. And who, you might ask, is watching to keep the nursing home honest? Most states require that clusters of new infections be reported to the local department of health. We are scrupulous about this and in most cases the office is helpful. It will even bend the rules on occasion if the greater good is served by doing so.

Now what about Tamiflu? When a cluster of the flu is noted and cases appear to be adding up, the practitioner at the home must decide whether to drop the bomb. Since, in most homes, one nursing unit will have several physicians, the infection control nurse and ultimately the medical director must make the call. If they are going to do it, they must do it quickly and decisively. It is a huge amount of work for that unit for that day, though if it stamps out the spread of the flu, it will save much more work down the road. The way orders are written in a home, every chart needs to have a new order written, every med sheet must be changed, and every order faxed to the pharmacy. Many units have at least fifty residents, so the work adds up. Add to that the need to actually give the extra doses of the medication for at least ten to fourteen days. No wonder many homes shy away from it, which is truly a pity. The greater pity, to put it all in perspective, is that some homes don't take prevention seriously enough.

The other major viral illness is the so-called viral gastroenteritis that is most often caused by the Norwalk Virus (part of a larger group known as Norvoviruses). Viral gastroenteritis can share the fever and muscle aches of influenza but results in nausea, vomiting, and diarrhea for up to five or six days. This is a daunting outbreak when it occurs. Our nursing home suffered an outbreak several years ago and it was devastating to residents and to staff. I caught it myself and can testify to its unpleasantness. Dehydration is rampant and many of our residents required intravenous fluids. There is no treatment; the virus runs its course. One must also prove that it's not an outbreak of food poisoning or even bacterial salmonella from the home's kitchen. To exclude that possibility, we usually culture two or three residents and report results to our local health department. Some labs can try to culture stool for the Norwalk Virus itself, but it can be as elusive as the Loch Ness monster.

Scabies and Other Bugs

Speaking of monsters, scabies is a disease of the skin that is caused by a fearsome-looking mite called *sarcoptes scabei*. Looking at it under the microscope can make your blood run cold. It looks like a horseshoe crab, but with gigantic, powerful claws. The whole bug is almost too small to see with the naked eye, but the eggs or "nits" are sometimes visible clinging to the hair of the abdomen, groin, or arms. Though it is associated with poor hygiene and can be found in homeless shelters, it can cause an outbreak in even the "best" and cleanest nursing homes. It is usually transmitted by a staff member or visitor and then takes up residence in the residents. It might stay in just one or two residents for a while and the team may mistake it for some other kind of condition, like eczema or dry, itchy skin. Without the proper treatment it will prove tenacious and the cause of much scratching and misery. It raises suspicion when other individuals and/or staff develop similar rashes and itching.

The implications are rather significant, which is why it is important to confirm whether scabies is present or not. The rash can be subtle, and unless the resident has a weak immune system, there may only be a few scratch marks and fewer than a dozen of the live little critters crawling around. In the old days, the primary-care doctor or a dermatologist would scrape the rash and look for the mite under the microscope. This is becoming a lost art and in questionable cases we call in a dermatologist to say yea or nay based on observation. Almost all homes have an outbreak every few years. The last time we had ours, it was fairly obvious what was going on.

Why are the stakes so high? It's not due to the treatment itself. One can use a cream called permethrin (Elimite), which is applied from the chin down to the toes (scabies in adults does not affect the face or scalp). After twelve hours, it is washed off and that often does the trick. If the mites or rash reappear or do not go away during the next week, we reapply the cream in the same fashion.

Another trick is to use an antiparasitic called ivermectin (Stromectol). This is a onetime oral dose of about 15–20 milligrams and I have had to resort to this a few times when the Elimite cream did not work. It is relatively safe, with rare liver toxicity, but has not been FDA approved for scabies.

The real hardship for the staff is that the mites continue to survive on bedsheets and clothes. These must be washed in very hot water and the staff must then place them in sealed plastic bags for several days. Bureaus and dressers must be examined for any hideaway clothes and then sealed as well so no clothes escape notice. Because this strategy usually ends up being applied to all residents on an affected unit, it is a Herculean amount of work, to say the least. That's why it is crucial to be sure or relatively sure of the diagnosis.

Bedbugs have made a comeback and even the ritzy hotel chains have been affected. There are some nursing homes that have had bedbugs and the key is to recognize the multiple bite marks on the residents and smears of blood on the sheets. The bedbugs fill up with blood and as the resident rolls over, she can crush a bug and crimson the sheet with blood.

Maggots are rare, but I have seen a few cases in different homes over the years. Maggots are simply the larvae of flies and look like tiny white worms. Usually the scenario is that a resident with an open wound is brought outside to get some sun by a staff or family member. Because she may be confused or have poor sensation over the wound area (as happens with diabetes), she will not sense a fly landing on the area and quickly laying some eggs. Within a day or two, the eggs turn into maggots and cause bleeding and tissue damage. Ironically, maggots are sometimes used medicinally to clean up infected or necrotic wounds, and the few cases I have seen bear this out. One must wash out and physically remove the maggots *or* one can cover the area with oil or paraffin.

Shingles

Another infectious curiosity that affects nursing home residents and is more common than maggots, scabies, and bedbugs combined is shingles. Shingles is the moniker for a condition known as herpes zoster, or just plain zoster. The reason for the name is that when it appears, little blisters are the hallmark of the rash and sometimes line up like shingles on a house. Shingles is an interesting story in its own right. The infection is actually a reawakening of the chicken pox virus (varicella zoster virus or VZV) that most people contract as children. Even though the rash goes away and the child recovers, the virus lies dormant in the nerve roots of the nervous system. In some people, the dormant virus never wakes up. In some, it comes out in times of stress or when the immune system weakens. It tends to reappear in advanced age, which is why in my nursing home of 300 people, we see at least 5 to 10 cases a year. About 15% of people who develop chicken pox will eventually have a case of shingles. More to the point, 50% of people over the age of eighty will have developed shingles at some point in their lives.

The most pressing concern in shingles is the acute and chronic pain that it causes. The acute episode varies from a small red rash with a few blisters to a whopping area with hundreds of tiny, painful blisters. The pain can even precede the rash by a few days. Clinicians have mistaken early shingles pre-rash for anything from heart attacks to inflamed gallbladders. Because the virus lodges in the nerve roots, when the rash blossoms it tends to follow the territory of a particular nerve root or "dermatome" emanating from the spinal cord. That is why we talk about the "dermatomal" location of an infection.

For example, the area of skin around the nipple is "supplied" by the fourth spinal root in the thoracic spine and is therefore known as the T-4 dermatome. This happens to be the same area that a heart attack may be felt and hence the confusion. A particularly vexing area to be involved is the cranial nerve that supplies the skin on the face and includes the eye. When the rash affects the eye, an ophthalmologist needs to be consulted quickly to determine the extent of the involvement. Sometimes the bark is worse than the bite and the eye itself is fine. Sometimes the covering of the eye (the cornea) can become inflamed, leading to scarring and blindness in that eye. This calls for special treatment and eyedrops and hence the need for an eye doctor. Another interesting characteristic of shingles is that it only occurs on one side of the body in that particular nerve area. If the rash crosses the midway point between right and left, it is unlikely to be shingles.

It is important to be as definitive as possible with a diagnosis because, as in scabies, the implications loom large. Shingles is potentially contagious, though nowhere near as much as chicken pox. Infection-control specialists recommend that only staff, visitors, and roommates who have had chicken pox be allowed in the same room as a resident with shingles. If for some reason a visitor or staff member who has not had chicken pox needs to care for a resident with shingles, he or she should wear a mask, gloves, and a disposable gown. Technically one needs airborne precautions as well, which is a whole other level of precaution involving negative pressure rooms. Nursing homes generally do not have these types of rooms, which is why we try to restrict access to only those who've already had chicken pox. Almost all elderly have had chicken pox, and thus we usually do not need to change rooms or roommates. If the roommate does not know or is immunosuppressed (most commonly from chemotherapy and/or cancer), then a room change is in order. Some directors of nursing always secure a private room for a resident with shingles, though it is not necessary.

Most residents with shingles heal in seven to ten days, at which point the staff can eliminate the precautions. Healing means that the lesions are crusted over and no fluid-filled blisters are visible. The rash may still be quite red and raw, but the key aspect is the state of the blisters (aka vesicles). Shingles almost never kills anyone, but there are two possible complications. If there is a lot of skin involved and there are open sores, a secondary bacterial infection known as cellulitis can occur. This can be severe and life threatening, and is usually accompanied by fever and a high white blood cell count. Many clinicians overreact to persistent redness by prescribing antibiotics. The other more dreaded complication is PHN or post-herpetic neuralgia. While the definition of PHN is controversial, it implies the persistence of pain in the area of the rash more than several months after resolution of the original rash. The older one is, the more common is the occurrence of PHN. The pain can vary from mild sensitivity over the affected area to completely disabling pain that has driven some to suicide. Caring for these individuals is challenging and treatments range from antidepressant, to antiepileptic, to narcotic medications. Most end up visiting a pain specialist, who sometimes performs injections to deaden the nerves and so seek to end the pain cycle. This meets with various levels of success.

Is there a medication that can treat the shingles and minimize the chances of developing PHN? Well, yes and no. Certain antiviral medications, the original of which was acyclovir, are active against the varicella zoster virus. The good news is that they will shorten the acute episode by a few days if given within forty-eight to seventy-two hours of onset. The bad news is that they by no means eliminate PHN. Some studies show that they do lower the chances of developing PHN and some show that they do not but that they shorten the length of time one suffers from PHN. In any event, the newer iterations of these medications have fewer side effects and can be taken fewer times per day. Nihilist though I am, I almost always think the risk/benefit calculation comes out in favor of treatment. I prescribe famciclovir (Famvir), though valacyclovir (Valtrex) is acceptable as well. It used to be standard to give a course of oral steroid medication, too, though this, based on more recent studies, has fallen out of favor.

Bacterial Illness and Multidrug-Resistant Bacteria (MDR)

Now let's forget maggots, scabies, bedbugs, and shingles and delve into the real heart of darkness—the world of multidrug-resistant bacteria. MDR bacteria have been in the news and with good reason: They represent a major threat to anyone in a hospital or nursing home. The root cause of these bacteria is the unrelenting use of antibiotics in the medical and agricultural world; the problem is worldwide and epidemic. We need first to appreciate some basics about bacterial infections. The most common bacterial infections in nursing homes occur in the lungs (pneumonia), in the urinary tract (UTIs), and skin (cellulitis).

Over one hundred years ago, the great medical thinker and professor Sir William Osler called pneumonia the "old man's friend." By that he meant that pneumonia was a graceful and welcome exit to the old and infirm in that era before antibiotics. Nowadays, pneumonia is eminently treatable. It is caused when the natural defenses of the body are overwhelmed and bacteria set up camp in a portion of the lung and multiply. Sometimes abnormal uncoordinated swallowing due to dementia or Parkinson's disease causes it; sometimes we cannot pinpoint the cause. Aspiration pneumonia is pneumonia caused by food or saliva from the mouth going down the wrong pipe into the trachea rather than the esophagus. The bacteria breed and attract cells from our own body that cause inflammation. The phlegm that often results is the residue of all this inflammation and signifies that the body is fighting the infection. It is also a sign, along with fever, shortness of breath, confusion, coughing, and a high white blood cell count, that pneumonia is brewing. In the frail nursing home resident, some of these signs and symptoms may be missing, but generally one or more is present.

Should the clinician suspect pneumonia, he or she would usually order the nurses to check the resident's vital signs more frequently, may order blood work to check for a high white blood cell count or signs of dehydration, and more than likely order a chest X-ray. A temperature check is part of the vital signs, but in the elderly, as with children, this is easier said than done. Many elders are mouth breathers and will not close their mouth over an oral thermometer to provide an accurate reading. Sometimes they are simply too confused to follow directions. The alternative is to take an axillary temperature, which means placing the thermometer under the armpit. If either the oral or axillary temperature is high (generally equal to or over 100 degrees Fahrenheit), that means there is a real fever. If it is normal or low, it may be a false negative. One caveat is that in cases of severe infection (sepsis), the temperature may be truly below 95 degrees. In any case, if the number does not match what the clinician thinks is going on, the proper thing to do is to check a rectal temperature. It pains me how rarely this is done and I can attest to the fact that an elevated rectal temperature has nailed down many a diagnosis in my practice that might otherwise have been missed. If your loved one *feels* warm despite a normal temperature reading, ask the nurse or nurse's aide to do a rectal temperature. They will generally oblige you; a doctor's order should not be necessary.

Chest X-rays in nursing homes are problematic at best. There are many mobile services in our area that perform chest X-rays within twenty-four hours of the request; they usually do them sooner than that but not always. Weekends, holidays, snowstorms, and hurricanes are tough... well, you get the picture. The battered mobile X-ray equipment can look like it served in a MASH unit during the Korean War. Add to that the fact that many nursing home residents cannot sit up properly or take a deep breath and you have the recipe for a mediocre test. The radiologist interpreters of the X-rays sit in remote offices like Greek oracles and, in my experience, rarely compare the present X-ray to a prior one. Older people often have abnormalities on their chest X-rays that have been present for years. Without comparing them to earlier films, the radiologist will often diagnose pneumonia that isn't there. In my nursing home, I have the ability to download the actual digital image on my computer and check the X-rays myself, but most facilities don't have that luxury.

It is not uncommon to see a *routine* admission X-ray read as "pneumonia" (or its code word "infiltrate") when the resident has no symptoms whatsoever. When the nurses call the doctor or, more likely, a covering doctor with the results, the path of least resistance is to prescribe antibiotics. If you care to be involved enough to monitor these scenarios, tell the home that you want to be *contacted for any change in medication*. The home should oblige by placing a note on the front of the chart to that effect. This can be a two-edged sword since they will now call you for everything, but these days, I'm not sure that's unwise. If you have had good experiences at the home and have no reason to suspect shoddy care, then let it ride. If you have had treatments begun that you questioned, or experienced a lack of communication, try to achieve some control through this mechanism. Certainly a change in your loved one with signs and symptoms of pneumonia coupled with an abnormality on a new X-ray spells pneumonia and treatment should start soon.

Urinary tract infection (UTI) is the other most common infection. The urinary tract is a long structure that begins in the penis or

vagina, encompasses the bladder, and then travels up the two ure-
ters, which are tubes connecting the bladder to each kidney. Infection of the lower tract generally involves the bladder and tends
to cause a mild fever, pain or burning on urination, the frequent
need to urinate, and cloudy and/or bloody urine. As the infection
climbs toward the kidneys, it can evolve into pyelonephritis, which
is marked by all of the above plus general malaise, loss of appetite,
higher fever, back pain, and even mental confusion. Since we are
talking about the elderly, some of these symptoms and signs may
be absent. Alternatively, the resident may have enough dementia
that she cannot express herself and the symptoms go unnoticed.
The accurate diagnosis of a UTI can be vexing indeed.

You may be asking what the difficulty is. Obtain a urine culture
and the diagnosis will be clear, right? Therein lies another rub.
When researchers performed studies on older people who had no
symptoms of a UTI and were not ill, about one-third had positive
cultures. When the population was checked several weeks later,
many of those with positive cultures had cleared and were negative whereas one-third of the previous negative cultures had turned
positive—again without anything to suggest a UTI! So cultures
are not the ultimate arbiter of a urinary infection. We call this
phenomenon of positive cultures without true infection "asymp-
tomatic bacteriuria." The positive culture means that the resident
is "colonized" but not infected; this concept rings true for other
infectious issues, as we shall see.

So what's a doctor to do? The best advice is to match up the
clinical picture with the culture data and be sure they jibe. The
corollary to this is not to check urine cultures without a reason
to do so—one will discover false positives, which invites the use
of unneeded antibiotics. Don't ask the doctor for "routine" cultures because your parent had a UTI in the past. I am also hesitant

when a nurse or family asks for a urine culture because there is a "foul smell" of urine in the room or because there is a slight change in mental acuity. These symptoms rarely correlate with real infection.

Some or most practitioners order a urine analysis (U/A) to go along with the culture. A U/A that is positive for leukocytes (white blood cells) can reveal inflammation in the bladder. I sometimes correlate this with the clinical picture and culture to help me determine if a true infection is present. Absent any signs of inflammation on the urine analysis and with few specific urinary symptoms, I am loath to treat a suspected UTI based on culture alone.

If all the data points to a true infection, then by all means antibiotics can help. The laboratory will usually send a second result a few days later called either a "biogram" or "sensitivity," which demonstrates to which antibiotics the bacteria are sensitive. In these days of resistant bacteria, it behooves the clinician to know these results and tailor the antibiotics when appropriate. I usually start with a sulfa (Bactrim or Septra) antibiotic or quinolone (Cipro or Levaquin, etc.) and await the biogram. If a culture shows two or more bacteria (some say three or more), it is unlikely to be an accurate reflection of an infection. Instead, it signifies contamination, which means the sample was not collected reliably and the urine was contaminated with the many bacteria that are found just outside the urethral area. We like to avoid catheterization (inserting a tube into the bladder via the urethra to collect a sample) due to the discomfort and the chance of causing bleeding or another infection. On occasion, though, when a resident is very sick or I am suspicious that there is a symptomatic UTI, I will order a catheterized specimen. This is especially true in a resident who is unlikely to cooperate, due to mental confusion, with catching a regular "clean-catch" sample.

Catheters raise another issue in long-term care. In the bad old days many if not most residents had permanent catheters in their bladders (sometimes known as Foley catheters). This was often for the convenience of the staff and represented a true hazard. These days, use of permanent catheters should be limited to the following situations: 1) The outflow of the urinary system is blocked and the resident cannot void without a catheter. In men, this is most often due to an enlarged prostate gland. In women, a blockage is less common but sometimes the bladder itself is weak and cannot generate enough "oomph" to void. If this situation persists despite attempts to rectify, the primary-care physician should consult a urologist. 2) The skin of the buttocks or backside has developed a pressure sore and the catheter keeps the area dry to promote healing in an incontinent resident. 3) The resident is nearing the end of her life and use of the catheter prevents unnecessary or painful moving of the resident.

From an infectious disease point of view, catheters are hall passes or conduits for bacteria and infection. Complicating the issue is that cultures from catheterized residents are almost always positive, meaning they grow bacteria. Remember my warning about colonization? The positive catheter samples, in the absence of signs and symptoms of infection, reflect colonization and should not be treated. By the same token, it is unwise and frankly bad practice to perform routine weekly or monthly cultures (unless there are highly resistant bacteria—see below). The practitioner should also not order a repeat culture after treating for a true infection, catheter or no catheter. The improvement in symptoms speaks for itself.

If the resident does not improve or gets frequent recurrent infections, it is worth obtaining a urologist's opinion. There may be a hidden blockage in the urinary tract or a bladder or kidney stone that is the breeding ground for repeat UTIs. I cared for a woman who was a Holocaust survivor and had had a truly miserable life. She had most recently had a stroke and was very difficult to understand, made worse by her frequent lapsing into Polish and her severe anxiety. She complained often of stomach pains. We finally understood them to be bladder pains with painful urination. We diagnosed her with a UTI and treated her, but she developed at least three more episodes over the next year. Because of her frequent complaints, many thought her to be crying wolf. Finally, the second urologist we consulted had the guts to perform a cystoscopy, which involved placing a small tube with a camera on the end into the bladder under anesthesia. He found not a hidden stone, but a suture that had been placed there years ago during some kind of operation. The suture had never been removed and was the source of her pain and infections. Removal of the suture improved her life and put an end to the infections. She was by no means perfect, but her life was made a bit more comfortable. Hats off to urologist #2 for taking the time that my patient deserved.

There remain a few other tricks for those with recurrent infection when no remediable cause can be found. Hygiene is critical. Staff must keep residents as clean as possible so that bacteria from bowel movements do not contaminate the urinary tract. Researchers have also found that intake of cranberries can reduce the frequency of UTIs: You may have already heard that as part of family lore and it appears to be true. Some nursing homes promote the ingestion of cranberry juice at mealtimes and some practitioners prescribe a concentrated form of cranberry extract in pill form. There is also a medication called methenamine (Urex, Hiprex, or Madelamine), which helps prevent bacteria from setting up camp in the bladder. It can be made even more effective by adding oral vitamin C, which adds acid to the urine and makes these medications more effective. Methenamine works in a different way from antibiotics and does not cause resistance.

Before we discuss resistant bacteria, there is one other infection that is the scourge of some nursing homes and hospitals: *Clostridium difficile* or *C. diff* for short. C. diff are among the many bacteria that live in and colonize the intestines. While it is capable of great harm, it is usually held in check by the millions of other bacteria in the gut. When the equivalent of a seismic jolt rocks the bacterial world of the intestines, the landscape of the gut changes and allows the C. diff to escape from its control by other bacteria. The seismic jolt in these cases is almost always an antibiotic. What we may see as the harmless use of antibiotics profoundly alters the ecology of the intestinal tract and allows the C. diff to reproduce wildly.

C. diff can cause severe inflammation of the lining of the large intestine with bleeding, diarrhea, crampy pains, and occasionally obstruction of the bowels and systemic infection. Years ago, this was unusual and gastroenterologists would often perform a sigmoidoscopy to look for the telltale pseudomembrane and so make the diagnosis of C. diff (aka pseudomembranous colitis). Nowadays, it is common enough that if the clinical situation fits and the resident was on antibiotics within the prior weeks to months, we send a stool sample for a C. diff assay. This test usually turns around in a day or two, but if my suspicion is high, I will start treatment and await the results.

The clinical picture of C. diff varies greatly; some residents develop a mild diarrhea while others are profoundly ill with high fevers and become dehydrated quickly. The test is only about 90% accurate, so even if it comes back negative but the clinical situation warrants, I will continue to treat for a full course. And what is the treatment? Paradoxically, the treatment is the same as the cause:

antibiotics. Even more paradoxically, the antibiotic we most often use has itself been on a few occasions the cause of C. diff. But let's leave that factlet for a medical Ripley's Believe It or Not.

The antibiotic now in favor to treat C. diff is metronidazole (Flagyl). It works best when taken orally though has some efficacy when given intravenously. It is also important to stop other antibiotics that may still be fueling the fire of C. diff colitis. The textbooks recommend treatment for ten to fourteen days. C. diff is a stubborn bug and often recurs despite treatment. Some experts retreat for a longer period with metronidazole and some switch to the alternative medication—oral vancomycin. While it is vital to attack the C. diff, we must also replenish other good bacteria as well. I generally give lots of yogurt or a probiotic such as acidophilus since some studies support this (though some experts do not feel that commercial yogurts or probiotic capsules contain many live bacteria). Some also use a cholesterol binder called cholestyramine (Questran) since it binds the toxic proteins that the C. diff produces and allows the normal bacteria to gain the upper hand. The danger of the binder is that it can bind other medications and must be given separately from them.

The key to preventing the spread of C. diff is hygiene and careful cleaning. Individuals with C. diff must be under contact precautions that are taken seriously. Contact precautions require gloves and possibly a disposable gown if one will be in contact with bodily fluids or material that might soil clothing. Still, hand washing is the single best deterrent to the spread of infection. While the alcohol-based gels and creams that are ubiquitous in some homes are great for ordinary bacteria, they are relatively ineffective against C. diff. Actual vigorous hand washing, including under the nails that lasts at least fifteen seconds, can dislodge the C. diff from one's hands. We recommend that the hand washer sing "Row, Row, Row Your

Boat" or the "Happy Birthday" song twice to be sure the cleaning lasts fifteen seconds. We also test the aides and nurses periodically to be sure they are following protocol.

I have to admit that my hand-washing skills have never been tested, but they should be. Recent studies demonstrated that doctors are the worst offenders; they often don't wash hands or don protective gear. Bacteria often contaminate their ties and stethoscopes. One of the deans warned us on the first day of medical school that we should look like the curers of disease, not the carriers of it! Of course he was referring to our sloppy dress, but the same applies to our cavalier attitude regarding infection control. If you are told that your parent has C. diff colitis and you do not find gloves and gowns outside the room for visitors and staff to wear, make a stink and demand that they do so.

C. diff forms spores that have been shown to survive on metal bed frames for months. The cleaning agent the nursing home uses must be able to kill these spores. Bleach-containing cleaners are the best. Our director of housekeeping is on our infection-control committee and each week receives a list of which residents harbor what infections. In that way, she can direct the staff to spend extra time and clean specifically against the infections at hand. Follow-up cultures are not necessary because it is almost impossible to eradicate the C. diff from the body; cultures may continue to be positive despite clinical recovery. Once the resident has "normal" formed stools (i.e., no diarrhea), the precautions can be removed. This does not give the staff carte blanche to ignore infection control; we still employ standard precautions, which afford protection but are a step down from contact precautions.

Precautions are also our best way to combat the new "alphabet soup" of multidrug resistant bacteria. MRSA, VRE, and ESBL are acronyms for bacteria that bedevil hospitals and have found their way into long-term care. The way a nursing home handles these infections speaks volumes about the quality of the home. You will likely not find a single hospital or nursing home in this country without them; they are omnipresent. The question is can the home manage these bacteria with as little disruption to daily life and as little risk to the residents as possible?

There is nothing especially virulent about these organisms; they are as harmful as their nonresistant counterparts. The catch is that once they are the cause of an infection, they are much more challenging to treat. Let's take the oldest of them, MRSA (methicillin-resistant staphylococcus aureus), which has been around since the late 1960s. Staphylococcus is related to the more familiar streptococcus of strep throat fame. Staphylococcus is a common cause of skin infections such as boils and is often the culprit in surgical wound infections. At first, all staphylococcus was sensitive to penicillin. As we used penicillin to treat it, resistance developed, but researchers came to the rescue with antibiotics such as methicillin, dicloxacillin, and some of its close cousins, the cephalosporins (like Keflex, etc.).

As we used these more and more (read *overused*), the crafty bacteria modified and mutated and became resistant, hence the handle methicillin-resistant. In fact, even many strep now are resistant to penicillin. Fortunately, we have come up with several antibiotics that can attack MRSA, such as vancomycin, linezolid (Zyvox), and daptomycin (Cubicin). Some of these must be given intravenously and some can be given orally, but either way, they cost a small fortune and the nursing home will often foot the bill for short-stay sub-acute residents. It is important to understand this because a home will often refuse to accept a patient from the hospital who is on one or more of these medications. It's hard to blame them since the daily cost of the drugs almost outstrips what

Medicare and insurance companies reimburse them. Interestingly enough, some of the MRSA are susceptible to older and cheaper antibiotics, such as sulfonamides (Bactrim and Septra) and tetracyclines. They are susceptible precisely because they are older antibiotics and no longer used enough to cause resistance.

This raises an important question. When the discharging doctor from the hospital writes an order for four weeks of Zyvox pills at $150 per day ($75 for each pill!), we better be darn sure the drug is necessary and that there are no alternatives. Hospital-based doctors—including specialists—are sometimes obtuse when it comes to cost. I frequently call them to discuss the need for the prescribed medications. When I tell them that the cost may interfere with their patient being treated (though at our home we take being nonprofit literally and often take the loss), they frequently come up with an alternative. Sometimes they admit that four weeks is overkill and shorten it to two weeks. Sometimes they convert to a cheaper but equally efficacious medication. Sometimes they admit that the infection may only be colonization and are willing to forego treatment.

Let's return to the C-word—*colonization*—that turns out to be central to our story. Because resistant bugs are ubiquitous, they often turn up when we perform cultures. If regular, plain-vanilla staph aureus lives in many people's throats or on their skin as colonizers, their pushy cousins the MRSA will show up as well. If we wouldn't treat run-of-the-mill staph aureus when there is no infection, then we should not treat MRSA either. This is a bit disingenuous; a gray zone exists. When we culture a pressure ulcer, for example, it will often grow bacteria such as MRSA. If the wound does not appear red or inflamed, or has no pus in it, and the resident has no fever, it is much more likely to be *colonized* than *infected*.

Two different clinicians can look at the same wound and opine differently. Some of the variation is based on experience. Some clinicians are trigger-happy and play the defensive medicine game; bedsores are fertile ground for malpractice lawyers. Whatever the reason, in many nursing homes and hospitals "mere" colonization is treated as infection and each round of antibiotics raises the ante for increased antibiotic resistance. Then again, we should not be getting cultures on wounds that don't *look* infected. Remember that C. diff colitis and disabling diarrhea often follow antibiotic use. Other side effects of antibiotics are legion but include rashes, nausea, and loss of appetite.

I should not direct my contempt only at my brother and sister physicians; they are not the only ones to blame. I receive at least one call a week from a family member to the tune of "You know, Mom sounds a little congested. Can you just give her some antibiotics?" I know you're concerned and maybe you think I would neglect your parent otherwise, but you're barking up the wrong tree. I'm afraid that calls like that *do* result in orders from other doctors for antibiotics over the phone without an examination. When I'm in a frisky mood and in a Clint Eastwood state of mind, I imagine myself fielding a call like this with a "Make my day, punk," and spouting off on the dangers of antibiotics. Don't get yourself in that situation. Just report what you are observing and ask me to see your mom.

Atul Gawande, the surgeon and medical author, wrote a review of Michael Moore's movie *Sicko* in *The New Yorker*. As much, he said, as we like to blame insurance companies for the failures in American health care, we should properly blame the American public. *It* has not yet shown by its wallets or by its votes that it is serious about reforming the system. So, too, on a smaller scale, the public's desire for antibiotics "just to be safe" is leading us down a dangerous path. I'm not exonerating the practitioner, but it takes two to tango.

The other two major resistant bacteria are VRE and ESBL. VRE stands for vancomycin-resistant enterococcus. This is a kind of bacteria that can cause a host of infections from pneumonia to urinary tract infections. Again, certain antibiotics like linezolid (Zyvox) are active against them; sometimes far cheaper and older medications still work. ESBL stands for extended spectrum beta lactamase-producing bacteria. These are bacteria that are highly resistant and tend to cause urinary and gastrointestinal infections. They are the latest to show up on the most wanted list and we are running out of antibiotics to use against them. The same caveats hold true for these as with the MRSA. Be sure the team is truly treating an infection and not colonization.

What is the natural history of colonization? Is there a way to treat someone who is colonized in order to eradicate the organism? If the resistant bacteria is causing an actual infection (not colonization) and the goals of the family are to treat, then the team needs to proceed with selecting an antibiotic that will work. This can be tricky because the information from the lab may be indecisive. It may report a bacterium as being *partially* resistant to a certain antibiotic or may not test another antibiotic that the practitioner might wish to try. In these cases, an infectious disease specialist *may* be helpful. It is rare that such a consultant will come to the nursing home but the primary-care provider may wish to consult over the phone or when he or she runs into that specialist at the hospital. The reason I say *may* be helpful turns on this point: Since the consultant may offer an opinion without ever laying eyes on the patient, he or she *may* offer only aggressive cookbook advice that is not in keeping with the reality of the person under treatment.

If your loved one is in his late nineties, has been treated three times for pneumonia resistant to almost all antibiotics, and suffers from advanced Alzheimer's disease, could it not be that pneumonia is visiting here as the "old man's friend"? I guarantee you that an infectious disease specialist will not comment on the ethical merits of the case or inquire as to whether a living will or health care proxy exists. He may suggest inpatient hospitalization with IVs and potent new antibiotics. Recall our discussion in chapter 9. Since your loved one may not recognize (due to dementia) that an IV is potentially helpful, he will end up restrained and catheterized. So first think clearly what your goals are—no, what his goals *would be*—and act accordingly. Don't let a slippery slope make you fall.

If the presence of MRSA, for example, represents colonization and the primary-care physician recognizes this (unfortunately a big "if"), then the proper course is to desist from further antibiotics. *The natural history is that the wound or urine or lungs will eventually "clear" the bacteria by themselves.* This can take one week or it can take one year. If the culture is from the urine and a catheter can be removed safely, the culture will become negative in short order. Thus have we "cleared" the colonization. On the other hand, I've been caring for a delightful woman named Millie who originally had a true eye infection known as conjunctivitis. We treated her for an MRSA infection with appropriate antibiotic eyedrops. The eye improved but the culture did not and enigmatically remained positive six months later. The eye was clearly colonized and the correct course of treatment after resolution of the infection was *not* to treat the colonization.

In most cases, the colonization would have cleared by itself, but with Millie, it did not. An eye specialist examined her to be sure there was not something abnormal in the eye that would cause her to retain the bacteria. There was not. Because Millie frequently touches her eye and has the capacity to spread the bacteria by hand, we even treated her one more time in an attempt to *eradicate* the bacteria. This was not successful.

Eradication has some fans, but many detractors. If a patient harbors resistant bacteria, has not cleared it spontaneously, and has the capacity to spread it to others, why not try once and for all to get rid of it? Not only does one give antibiotics, but the practitioner tries to find the region(s) of the body that is harboring the bacteria. This is most often the nose, but sometimes the rectum or both. This is why we sometimes do cultures from these areas and include them in treatment protocols if they are positive. Most commonly we apply an ointment called mupirocin (Bactroban) to the nostrils for a prolonged period of time. For good measure and using a car-wash mentality, some throw in a series of baths or showers using a special detergent called chlorhexidine with which surgeons sometimes scrub before surgery. Eradication sounds good in theory, but the colonization generally recurs.

And how do we know that? In contrast to the situation with C. diff, we *do* perform follow-up cultures on anyone with MRSA, VRE, or ESBL. This determines when the contact precautions can be suspended. As long as the cultures remain positive, we maintain precautions. The protocol recommended by most infectious disease specialists is that we require two negative MRSA cultures within a forty-eight- to seventy-two-hour stretch to pronounce someone clear of MRSA. With VRE, we ask for three weekly negative cultures. ESBL is a bit up in the air. In our home, we go by the MRSA rules. The precautions, for the most part, are contact precautions. Some homes place these residents in a private room and have them eat by themselves, too. We need to balance such limiting and restrictive measures against the resident's rights and needs to move freely through the home.

For example, Millie loves the music programs on Thursday afternoons and the bingo games on Tuesdays. Can we really deprive her of these events because she is on contact precautions?

We have creatively arrived at an individual care plan that balances all these considerations and it's no easy task. Millie is allowed to go to certain events where we can keep a good eye on her and her interactions with others. She sits alone to eat but is close enough to others to participate in a conversation. My guess is that none of the other residents know of her condition; we do what we can to protect her privacy.

Millie is relatively easy because she has a basic understanding of her condition. Residents with dementia are another matter. They are unable to observe precautions that require active cooperation from the resident. How does one maintain residents largely in their room when they don't always recall where their room is? How do you ensure that they do not touch other residents? *Don't ask, don't tell* doesn't exactly work well here.

Should we be testing all residents for drug-resistant bacteria? Recent research from the University of Pittsburgh hospital's ICU may be suggestive. Like almost all intensive care units in the country, more than two-thirds of their patients tested positive for multidrug-resistant bacteria. The good news is that by zealously identifying these patients and isolating them with proper precautions, they lowered the rate of resistant bacteria to less than 20%. This makes a strong case for "surveillance" cultures of everyone in a health care setting such as an ICU. Does it also apply to the nursing home? While it may seem obvious, we don't know the answer. In our imperfect nursing home world we try to maintain precautions and to culture frequently those we have identified, but we do not perform surveillance cultures on all residents (which would ideally include staff as well). The expense would be significant both in the testing and the labor involved. Stay tuned as this problem evolves; it is finally on the politicians' and the public's radar screen.

Can a home refuse to admit a patient who harbors one of these bacteria? These days the answer is mostly no, but a small dose of history may be helpful. When I was in training in the mid-1980s and multidrug-resistant bacteria were not as common, very few nursing homes would accept a patient who tested positive. They demanded that the patient have negative cultures before accepting them in transfer. That was also a time when waiting lists for nursing homes were long and they could afford to be choosy. In order to get a patient out of the hospital, we did just what we now advise clinicians not to do: We treated colonization with antibiotics and this, in turn, bred more resistance. Nowadays, positive cultures for MRSA, VRE, and ESBL are so common, and so many homes have open beds, that acceptance is the norm and the nursing homes "deal." They know that if they turn someone down, the home down the street will say yes. The accepted resident should have a plan of care and if that home insists on a private room, you may need to wait until a private room presents itself. This can explain the persistence of some "delays" when it comes to nursing home transfers. The homes that accept many patients straight out of the hospital for sub-acute care will be the ones with the highest rates of these resistant bacteria. When these rates are published as some states have legislated, some families will be scared needlessly—others appropriately. What one needs to know is that the home takes infection control seriously, has an active infection-control committee, and enforces precautions strictly but with a heart, as in Millie's case.

12

The Final Chapter:
End-of-Life Care

"As long as Mom can still smile, we'd like to keep her around as long as we can." So went the response of one of my patient's sons when I asked him about his goals for his very ill mother, Dotty. Let me back up. Almost every day I confront the issue of end-of-life care with a patient or a family member—that's just the nature of my job.

When I'm stymied and I feel that I'm not getting my point across, I ask what I've been trained to ask. I want the son or daughter or patient to sum up for me succinctly what's most important at this, the last stage of life. I try to have the family erase for a moment all the factual questions having to do with X-rays, blood counts, medications, fevers, and prognoses. I want them to focus on the intangibles, the low-tech question of what would be most important to the quality of one's life. I ask very simply, "What are your goals for your mom as she enters this difficult but final stage of her life?" Almost always, the answer is something like "please just keep her comfortable" or "just be sure she's not in any pain." This gives me an opening to give them my opinion about how we can assure that aim and transcend some of the questions that obfuscate that goal. It doesn't always work, as you can tell by the response of Dotty's son.

Dotty had a severe stroke four years ago that left her paralyzed on one side of the body. She had never been a very active person but slipped into a sedentary existence at our nursing home. She was completely dependent on the staff to get her out of bed, help her bathe, and dress. She had occasional infections and with each episode, she emerged more dependent. About four months before this conversation, she developed a blockage in her kidneys from kidney stones and was hospitalized for a systemic infection. We treated her aggressively; she did not have a living will and her two sons wished all measures taken to ensure her survival. She managed to survive by dint of powerful antibiotics and a tube placed in the conduit from one of her kidneys to her bladder that temporarily relieved the blockage.

The combination of the illness and the anesthesia for the procedure hit her hard. On her arrival back at the home, she lost most of her ability to speak except to repeat her name or say simple phrases like "I'm fine." Her appetite flagged and she lost over twenty pounds in the next three months. She developed a sore that would not heal on her left leg (her circulation and diabetes saw to that). She was a shell of her former self. Her smile sometimes shined through and this, more than anything, was what her sons noticed.

After three months, the tube that the urologist placed needed to be changed (under anesthesia again) for fear of infection and Dotty was living on borrowed time. The urologist was reluctant to proceed given her frailty and the risks that surgery and anesthesia would entail. I spoke with the sons many times and they could not come to grips with making a decision about the procedure. One brother said he was going to call the other and vice versa. Do not misunderstand. These are two of the most caring and able sons you would care to meet. Sometimes, though, if you don't quite kill with kindness, you can come close.

The sons did eventually contact the urologist, who painted an accurate picture for them. As bad luck would have it, Dotty developed a high fever and quickly became dehydrated. I was away at the time, but my covering physician admitted her to the hospital where she again received aggressive care and the urologist changed the tube to quell the infection that had lodged in it. She survived once again, but could not hold her head up and coughed whenever we tried to feed her. She did not seem to reliably follow anything I asked her, like "raise two fingers on your hand." She did at times show more awareness around her sons and could motion to them or refer to them as her sons. Her quasi smile stuck to her as if painted on; it looked like one-quarter smile to three-quarters grimace.

I could not keep Dotty in the hospital any longer. Her fever and infection had abated and she accepted food if spoon-fed to her by the staff and family. She was weak as a kitten and seemed to me to be only days away from another infection or pneumonia. She had developed a bedsore on her bottom after only being in the hospital for a week. I spoke to the sons several times by phone and sat down with them at the bedside. As we say in the profession, I laid plenty of "crepe" and told them she was getting close to the end. I told them she was crossing over to the side of suffering and, if it were my mom, I would opt for hospice care and keep her at the nursing home from then on. She would only continue to lose weight and the sores on her bottom and leg would not heal.

The sons were pretty sure they did not want an artificial feeding tube, though asked me several questions over and over again. The questions mostly touched on the technical and they could not come to grips with the idea of comfort care. I knew Dotty would die (as much as anyone can "know" this) and would suffer if we pursued aggressive care. It was then that I posed the question about "goals."

The sons did not take the bait and instead of talking about comfort and wanting their mom to be out of pain, they could only talk about "keeping her around." And why? The smile that had gotten Dotty through the Great Depression might now be her undoing. The sons told me that as long as she could smile and recognize them, they would want me to treat aggressively to keep her alive.

As I write this, Dotty has been back at the nursing home and barely holding her own. She's completing the last days of her antibiotics and is back on intravenous feedings because her intake is so poor. The sons, who only think they are doing right by their mom, ask me for daily phone conferences about Dotty's status. I feel like I've said it all and I'm running out of words. Will I have any words of comfort when that time really comes? Dotty's story is real and repeats itself daily in homes, nursing homes, and hospitals throughout this country.

Let's define some terms. The problem that permeates end-of-life care in our country is a lack of planning. No one wants to think about the end, but it is necessary. Planning ahead to be sure your wishes are followed is known as "advanced care planning" and is elemental in our discussion. As a society we have traveled light-years in the last decade, but we still have far to go. The federal government enacted the Patient Self-Determination Act of 1990 in order to allow and encourage people to participate in their own health care decisions. Since 1990, every health care facility that receives federal funding (essentially all facilities) has been required to provide information on how to plan for future health care contingencies. You need *not* wait until you are in a health care setting.

Most lawyers have serviceable forms; one can even buy them on the Internet from reputable sites such as Americans for Better Care of the Dying at www.abcd-caring.org.

Advanced care planning includes two principal documents. The first is the living will. There are many iterations of this document and there is no standard that is used throughout the country. The living will allows you to state, in the event that you become seriously ill and can no longer make your own decisions, what kind of treatment you want and how aggressive you want that treatment to be. Some living wills are specific and some are vague. They all allow you to specify whether you would wish to forego CPR (cardiopulmonary resuscitation) and/or other medical treatments in the event that you need it. I will discuss CPR and other acronyms like DNR later in this chapter. For now, suffice it to say that living wills can prohibit the practitioner from using artificial feeding tubes or intravenous hydration (which many of my patients have told me they would not want) if the time comes. One can also include dialysis, antibiotics, surgery, or whatever you feel you would not wish to have performed on you. If you are aware and alert when these decisions arise later in your life, you can certainly make those decisions at the time. The purpose and genius of the living will is that there may come a time when you *cannot* make those decisions but still want your wishes to be observed. They can be painstakingly specific and list all kinds of different scenarios. My advice is to be specific but keep it relatively simple so your doctors will read the darn thing. Some lawyers write them free-form and can really spell out what you do or don't want.

Completing this in *advance* is important because it allows decisions to be based on the values that you cherish without a medical team forcing an answer in the heat of the moment. I have witnessed too many scenes like this: An elderly and frail ninety-something from a nursing home with progressive dementia arrives in the ER with a heart attack and labored breathing. As they connect her to a heart monitor, the team sees that she is minutes away from a cardiac arrest. The future for this person, if she survives, will be bleak due to the advancing dementia. Had she thought about it years ago, she might have told her daughter or best friend, "If I ever get to the point where I don't recognize you and have little pleasure in life, please just let me go."

Unfortunately, nothing was ever written down and in the heat of the moment, the daughter either is absent or doesn't remember the discussion. Even if she is present and *remembers* the discussion, the medical team in the ER might say something like "Do you want us to do everything we can to save your mom or should we do nothing and just let her go?" It takes a pretty tough and self-confident daughter (or son) to face down the medical team in these situations and insist on doing nothing. Would that the doctors had taken a class on communication and sensitivity. In many ERs the doctors' concern is liability; they are more afraid of undertreating than overtreating. ERs are fast-paced places and the doctors who inhabit them make decisions quickly because they have to. The moral of the story is to be sure an advance directive such as a living will exists and that it comes over from the nursing home.

Some living wills carry verbiage that can be vague at best and confusing at worst. The language often reads, "If two physicians have determined that I am in a terminal state with no reasonable expectation of survival, then do not place me on life-support machines and do not perform CPR." The problem with this language is how to define "terminal state" or "no reasonable expectation of survival." It is rare in a nursing home that I am treating someone with cancer who truly has only weeks to live. The more typical case is a resident with progressive Alzheimer's disease or severe emphysema for whom medication is no longer working. Many laypeople and lawyers do not consider these to be terminal states. More appropriate verbiage would reflect the person's position on the continuum of life such as no longer recognizing family and friends, not eating enough to sustain oneself, or being so sedentary that bedsores have developed. Living wills are beginning to reflect this change in attitude.

The other important document is a health care proxy, durable power of attorney for health care, or something that sounds similar. In these documents, the individual designates one other person (sometimes with an alternate) to make health care decisions if she becomes unable to make them herself. You may think this is redundant if a living will already exists. Living wills sometimes cannot be found or the reading of them is unclear. A proxy ensures that the health care team follows the person's wishes. Needless to say, the proxy should be someone the individual trusts literally to the end of time. The proxy is usually a spouse or child but sometimes is a friend, a clergy member, or even a physician. What if, as happens on occasion, the health care proxy contradicts the living will? Children especially feel guilty or want the "best care that money can buy" and go against a living will. They may even claim that the living will was not valid.

I took care of a woman several years ago who was in the throes of dying. She was truly terminal. We read her living will and it was ironclad that she did not want heroic measures, such as feeding tubes, resuscitation, or even hospitalization. We informed the family, which consisted of a daughter and a son-in-law. They were furious with us that we would not seek the most aggressive care possible and wanted her shipped immediately to the local ER. We wanted to do right by this woman and ferreted out the designated health care proxy.

Sure enough, the patient had *not* designated her own daughter as her proxy but listed her family physician, who for years had taken care of her on the outside. The fact that she bypassed her own daughter was unusual and significant. The daughter and son-in-law were deeply religious and had a fundamental objection to limiting care, even if it meant opposing the mother's wishes. I immediately notified our administrator of the conflict, sat through a very stormy session with the daughter and son-in-law, and enlisted our local ethics advisory committee to visit and make comments.

Ethics committees are sometimes homegrown in the nursing home or hospital; we had the benefit of a county group that was able to come the same day. The members of the committee supported the patient's advance directive. More important, we tracked down her family physician, who was on a beach at the Jersey shore enjoying his retirement. He confirmed, with a remarkable memory for the facts, that the woman deliberately did *not* want her daughter making decisions because of divergent values and beliefs. He was only too glad to fax us a letter (after he got off the beach) reaffirming the advance directive and the patient's wishes. We still had to stare down the family and weather the threat of a lawsuit. The process took hours and plenty of spine. I'm sad to say that many facilities would have given in to the family. We were fortunate indeed that the family physician also wanted to do the right thing.

Proxies *are* important. You or your parent should sit down with the proxy and be sure he or she understands exactly what the living will states *and* that you want it honored. The best living wills have a statement that admonishes the reader to follow it *even if* the proxy or family disagrees. Now, just because there is a living will and/or a proxy does not mean that the medical orders in the nursing home chart reflect that. The physician still must translate the living will into an order such as a DNR (Do Not Resuscitate). That usually follows a discussion with the physician (or nurse practitioner) as to what advance directive is in place. Some homes designate a social worker to have the discussion and report that to the physician. There are many homes in this country that still do not specify orders even when an advance directive is completed and available. Be sure that your parent has an advance directive, that a copy of it is in the chart, and that you have discussed with the practitioner orders such as a DNR if that is what you choose.

DNR is the first of the three "Ds" in advance care planning. If a patient is DNR, she will not receive maximal efforts (CPR) to bring her back to life if found not breathing and without a pulse. Hmm…not breathing and no pulse? What's the difference between that and being dead? It's probably about the same as the difference between the naked and the nude, which is to say it depends how you look at it, but not much difference at all. A medical ethicist named Dr. Michael Gordon from Toronto has written compellingly on the subject. Tongue in cheek, he even suggests that the "R" in DNR stands for resurrection because resuscitation is all but futile in nursing home residents.

Resuscitation comprises CPR and more advanced life support with medications, defibrillation, and ventilator assistance. It was developed in the early 1960s for patients who suffered a "witnessed" cardiac arrest as sometimes happens in the middle of a heart attack. CPR was used to continue the flow of blood and oxygen to the brain and body while medications and ventilation were used to get the heart beating again. Even with CPR, after five to ten minutes of limited circulation, the brain begins to suffer damage that is accentuated in the highly susceptible brains of the elderly.

Results of resuscitation attempts are notoriously disappointing in nursing home residents. Dr. Gordon summarizes the results in a paper that appeared in the *Annals of Long-Term Care* in 2003 entitled "CPR in Long-Term Care: Mythical Benefits or Necessary Ritual?" Several large studies have shown dismal results of resuscitation in nursing home residents. Of four hundred attempted resuscitations in three different studies, there were only *two* survivors, one of whom died eight months later, malnourished and with a large and painful bedsore.

Most cardiac arrests in nursing homes are unwitnessed. When the resident *is* discovered, she has in all likelihood been dead for hours. Many homes do not perform resuscitation and rely on the local first-aid squad to get to the building and administer it. You may ask, "Why not at least give CPR a shot so I can be sure everything was done?" The answer to that resides in the adage, "a picture is worth a thousand words." Though it was not invented to inflict pain, resuscitation in a frail older person is a near-violent process that frequently fractures ribs and the breastbone due to forceful chest compressions. Large needles are inserted in the groin and neck to administer medications and fluid. A breathing tube is inserted (read *rammed*) down the throat to try to deliver oxygen. This can go on for ten to twenty minutes and is antipodal to death with dignity.

I have been on the administering end of CPR many times. All too often these have been in the unfortunate cases when a family didn't "get it" and did not consent to a DNR. I would gladly have been anywhere else in the universe. I think that if families could see what was being inflicted on their loved one, they would scream "DNR" from the hilltops. The fault, though, resides as much with my profession for not sitting down with families and telling it like it is.

When a DNR is ordered, the facility often requires a physician or nurse practitioner to document and explain in the chart that they spoke with the patient and/or family. In most states, this conversation can even take place on the phone. It should be with the health care proxy (or legal guardian in the cases where one exists) but *can* be with the next of kin (usually the person who takes financial responsibility for the resident and signs her into the home). The courts have not wanted to be in the business of determining who can and cannot give consent to an advance directive. Unless someone challenges it legally, it will stick. In New York and perhaps in other states, the rules are stricter and the patient or family must sign a DNR form, too.

The ability to obtain a DNR depends very much on how it is "sold" to a family or resident. In my experience, residents who can make decisions for themselves are much quicker to agree to a DNR than are their children. Many of my residents have lived a long and full life. They mostly are familiar with living wills. It is *their* body and they are most fearful of living compromised, dependent lives. They also, frankly, don't want to experience the pain of being on a machine or feel the pain of CPR. "I've lived long enough," "I don't want to be a burden," and "If I went to sleep tonight and didn't wake up, it would be fine with me" are the most frequent comments I hear.

Children sometimes have a tougher time. In general, families with less education or who are angry at the system, and who have not heard about living wills, are less likely to agree to a DNR. Language barriers can make discussions a challenge and it is worth obtaining a translator. While I always present DNR as an *option*, I suppose I could be accused of gilding the lily. Because of my experiences and because of the dismal results of CPR, I give my opinion freely. If a resident is relatively healthy and vigorous, I present the options without editorializing. These residents, though, are fewer and further between. I often ask them to think about any other family member who might have been gravely ill and ended up on a ventilator or had a miserable final stay in the hospital. Families often cite these experiences to *me* when choosing a DNR. If it seems clear that the burden of aggressive care and resuscitation far outweigh any benefit, I will say something like "I'm going to assume, given your mom's overall situation, that you would not want her to be placed on life support if it came to that." I usually know my audience because families almost always agree. For some families it is so hard to make the call and to live with the guilt that I'm happy to take that responsibility off their shoulders. Just so you know I'm playing fair, I always clarify at the end about what we've spoken and what a DNR means. Too many doctors don't share their opinions and experiences. In an effort to avoid being paternalistic or simply to avoid liability, they either eschew the topic or present it in such a light that families feel "guilted" into maximal, high-tech aggressive care.

DNR means no CPR, no ventilator (artificial breathing machine that supplies ventilation through a tube in the windpipe), and no electric shock (defibrillation) in the event of a cardiorespiratory arrest. DNR does not mean "Do Not Care"; many people inside and outside the profession hold this misconception. DNR simply expresses the wish of a patient not to undergo heroic measures. When DNRs first came on the scene, they were used only for people who were hours or days away from death and the DNR label did signify "no care." Nowadays, DNRs are common in nursing homes and hospitals. A DNR patient and/or his family may still request aggressive care short of heroics. Some living wills may preclude treatments like antibiotics, but a DNR by itself does not. Families occasionally decline a DNR because they think their loved one will be ignored or that we will give up. I assure them that this is not the case. Through education, I think we are winning the battle.

The second "D" is DNI or Do Not Intubate (i.e., do not place on a ventilator). The end of life is not always sudden. A resident may decline steadily such that she can no longer sustain her breathing but her heart has not stopped and she is not in arrest. For these situations, which most often happen in a hospital, some facilities identify the DNI option. Some hospitals do not offer this and assume a DNR always precludes intubation. The staff may ask you to further clarify a DNR by signing or not signing a DNI. Think carefully about it. Most residents who require a ventilator to survive have severe underlying disease and their chances of dying or being placed back on a ventilator in the next few weeks to months are very high.

Ventilators are painful and frightening machines. The patient is usually so agitated and resistive to the machine that she needs to be heavily sedated or chemically paralyzed. The weaning process can be very slow and in the elderly is complicated by generalized weakness.

Ventilators carry risks, too. They frequently trigger pneumonia with resistant bacteria (known as a nosocomial or hospital-acquired infection). If the doctors cannot wean the patient from the ventilator within seven to ten days, a tracheostomy may be necessary. Instead of the tube to the ventilator passing through the mouth and the throat, it goes directly through an opening in the windpipe or trachea. So if you agree to intubation, do so with the knowledge that things can get "real" in no time flat. Doctors have a way of talking you into something that may seem trivial to them but can have dire and agonizing consequences. They may say, "Let's try it for a while and see how it goes." Sounds great in theory, but in practice if your parent doesn't improve, it's emotionally tougher to remove the ventilator than not to begin down that road in the first place.

The third "D" is DNH and stands for Do Not Hospitalize. Some nursing homes now recognize that many residents and their families wish their loved ones to be "treated in place," which means *in* the nursing home. For all the reasons we have discussed, they wish to forego hospitalization. This does not connote that they wish no treatment: IV antibiotics, X-rays, and frequent practitioners' visits *can* happen at many nursing homes. A DNH does mean that if someone is so sick that they might die, they will be allowed to die with dignity at the home, in friendly environs with particular attention to comfort and the palliation of symptoms. How's that for loading the dice? A painless passing, surrounded by loved ones and staff that have become a second family—can it really happen? A late-day Lazarus, I've seen it with my own eyes and not just once.

What if a nursing home either does not offer DNH or you question whether there is enough staff so that your loved one is not left to suffer in silence? The answer may be hospice. Even in better homes, hospice can offer services that should put your mind at ease.

Hospice was started in England in the early 1960s to help ease the passing at home of people with terminal diseases. It has spread throughout the world and now almost half of the hospice care in this country is provided in nursing homes. The federal government estimates that 10–15% of nursing home residents meet criteria for hospice. The actual utilization of hospice is far less. I have described in earlier chapters what hospice provides and in the case of my patient Bertha—discussed in chapter 9—how valuable it was in her care. The nursing home must have a contract with hospice and any good-quality home will have one if not more.

Some homes are reluctant to let a resident die in the facility. This is a vestigial view from the days when nursing homes sent anyone legitimately sick to the hospital. Some homes also try to maximize their revenue by caring for a resident who returns from the hospital at a higher Medicare reimbursement rate. Most homes thankfully have moved beyond these approaches. If you wish a comfort DNH approach, enlisting hospice may be the ace up your sleeve. Some doctors are still misinformed that hospice is only for cancer patients in whom death is imminent. Still others "don't believe in it" (do they not "believe" in death either?). You can usually work around the doctor if that's the case by talking to the social worker or the administrator of the home. If that still does not work, you might want to find the name and number of the hospice that takes care of residents at your parent's nursing home. Ask to speak to the intake coordinator and explain the situation. If that leads nowhere and you feel the facility is violating your loved one's rights, then crack open your Rolodex and call your state ombudsman.

Medicare and most insurers pay the cost and hospice provides extra benefits, such as nurses who ensure that the resident is comfortable. The resident generally remains in her own room unless the home happens to have a separate hospice unit (which is rare). Hospice can also provide one-on-one nursing assistants for several hours a day. The aide should help feed the resident and provide more care than the home could otherwise provide. The family can help determine what is the best use of the aide's time.

We have, from time to time, observed the "hospice phenomenon." Some residents with advancing dementia develop weight loss from a combination of poor appetite and lack of ability to feed themselves. If this continues and the medical team has excluded other causes of weight loss, the resident may meet criteria for hospice. The doctor has to certify that if the dementia (or other disease) runs its natural course, the resident will likely die within six months. Even though the nursing home needs to provide someone to help feed the resident, that staff member may also be feeding four other residents. A one-on-one hospice aide can be far more attentive and efficient and we have seen some of these residents gain weight and, in time, "graduate" from hospice. Hospice will usually dismiss the resident within a few months of the weight loss reversal; the resident can always reenter hospice if the decline recommences.

Hospice also shifts the focus away from aggressive care, lab numbers, and X-rays to what most agree is more important: your loved one's ability to spend as much time before she dies in the company of family and friends in a calm and soothing environment. There are pastoral services and social work services beyond what the home can usually provide. The hospice nurses also speak with the physicians directly with any advice or suggestions about pain control and to ameliorate symptoms that might attend the dying process.

Competency and Decisional Capacity

In discussing advance directives, I mentioned that they don't take effect until the older person loses the ability to make decisions. How does one decide when a resident of a home (or any older person) loses the ability to make decisions? There are several terms that are tossed around that we need to clarify. Competency is a legal decision made by a court. If someone is competent, then he or she can attend to the ordinary affairs of life, such as shopping, clothing, managing finances, and paying bills. People are presumed competent unless there is evidence to the contrary. In older people with dementia there is often evidence against competency and the judge can decide that a legal guardian is needed. The judge will incorporate the reports of two practitioners when making a decision. These reports can be from psychiatrists, psychologists, or regular physicians. Guardianship is usually not necessary when there is family around that is willing to take responsibility. This is a gross simplification since other legal mechanisms like durable powers of attorney exist that allow access to bank accounts and other personal information.

What we are more concerned with in long-term care is capacity or really decisional capacity. In other words, can the person make informed decisions? They don't have to be "good" decisions or decisions that you or I might make. To have decisional capacity, the person must understand what is being asked, be able to comprehend the consequences of accepting or rejecting care, and can repeat back or explain what she has been told and what she has decided. Capacity is not decided by a court or a judge, but by a practitioner. The practitioner is often the physician of record who receives input from the care team. I may think that I know my patients well but "stuff happens" and the resident may not be the person I remember. I ask the nurses and aides key questions first and then sit down with the resident to ask my own questions.

If it's pretty clear-cut, I can stop there and usually jot a note in the chart. If not, I may ask a psychiatrist or another physician for a second opinion. Capacity need not be global; capacity can be decision specific. Even if a resident has early Alzheimer's disease, she may understand what it means to be on life support and has even thought about it before. Her wish for a DNR order may be perfectly reasonable and based on capacity to make her own decisions about health care. The same resident may not be able to understand the intricacies of cancer treatment options; for that, we would turn to a living will or the family.

Family members don't always agree, but usually we can come to an accord in a family meeting. In a typical case, three out of four children will agree on a DNH, but the last one disagrees, wants to be heard, and needs more time. Sometimes the last one *refuses* to go along with the group. If one of the others is the health care proxy, he or she can rule the day. In my experience, most children like to have everyone on board and of the same mind. Each family is different and has its own dynamic. Sometimes a good social worker working with the family and the care team can bring closure and agreement. Rarely does the situation disintegrate into conflict and legal challenge.

New Approaches to Advance Directives

The advance directive structure is fragmented. Some nursing homes and hospitals are stricter than others and have stringent policies while others leave it more to chance and the vagaries of the different physicians. Different states have different rules. Some ambulance companies and EMTs honor a DNR from a nursing home and some do not. A national movement has crystallized that seeks to standardize the process. It originated in Oregon in 1991 and is slowly spreading throughout the country. It is known in some parts as POLST (Physician Orders for Life-Sustaining Treatment) and in other parts as MOLST (Medical Orders for Life-Sustaining Treatment). POLST/MOLST is an effort to have one set of advance directives that is standard, self-explanatory, easy to read, follows the person through the health care maze, and is accepted by nursing homes, hospitals, and EMTs alike.

A state has to endorse the form before it must be accepted by facilities in that state. Not all states have signed on yet. For example, New York has endorsed the MOLST while New Jersey has not. Not all facilities or practitioners in New York are familiar with MOLST, but in time one hopes they will be. The MOLST/ POLST encapsulates the major issues of resuscitation, intubation, artificial nutrition, and hydration on an attractive hot pink foldout form and is signed and reviewed periodically by the practitioner. Copies can be made to accompany the patient to other health care venues such as hospitals and outpatient centers. It's our best hope right now to establish a coherent, legal, and effective means to honor someone's health care wishes.

Artificial Nutrition and Feeding Tubes

One of the points that almost all living wills address is artificial feeding. Unless someone dies suddenly from a heart attack or massive stroke, chances are they will reach a point of not being able to nourish their own bodies. Advanced dementia is perhaps the clearest example and behaves somewhat like cancer. We think of cancer as a terminal illness and the loss of appetite and weight as defining the last stages of the disease. Dementia, too, culminates in a loss of the cues for hunger and thirst. The victim also loses the physical ability to hold a spoon and to grip a glass, and this combination results in dehydration and loss of weight. Severe heart disease, Parkinson's, multiple sclerosis, and emphysema are but a few of the other diseases that conclude with this picture. This is essentially the way humans died for millennia before the advent of artificial feeding. Let's put off a discussion of the ethics of artificial feeding until we understand the mechanics of it.

The first most temporary means by which to feed a patient artificially is the nasogastric tube. A nurse or doctor at the bedside places this flexible plastic tube through the nose, down the back of the throat, and into the stomach. It is uncomfortable, but in experienced hands takes only a minute or two. Some patients resist and others are very sensitive in which cases it takes more like ten to twenty minutes. The tubes can be used to deliver artificial feedings for up to two weeks, at which point they can cause erosion of tissues and need to be removed.

For several reasons, nasogastric tubes are not very practical in nursing homes. Even if they were easier to place, the tubes are so annoying to people that they mostly try to pull them out. Hospitals routinely restrain people by tying their hands to the side of the bed; nursing homes by regulation should not be doing this. Ethically, it is very hard to justify prolonging a life by tying someone down, fastening her to a bed, and causing complications like bedsores and pneumonia.

Since the end of the nineteenth century, surgeons have experimented with a tube placed directly via surgery through the abdominal wall into the stomach to deliver nutrition. The original goal was to provide a surfeit of calories to patients after serious surgery and/or trauma. These gastrostomy tubes can still be used effectively for that purpose and are removed when patients have recovered to the point where they can feed themselves. At some point physicians began using gastrostomy tubes for older people who could no longer nourish themselves. The development of a nonsurgical technique to place these tubes in the early 1980s dramatically altered the scene and complicated the ethical debate.

The PEG (percutaneous endoscopic gastrostomy) tube can be placed by a nonsurgeon (usually a gastroenterologist) in a matter of twenty minutes or less. It is a procedure rather than a full-scale operation and does not require an operating room. It is performed in the endoscopy suite and requires only sedation rather than general anesthesia. It is not risk-free, but is safer than the placement of surgical tubes. That's a good thing, because the procedure is performed on the frailest of the frail usually after a life-threatening illness in demented patients. The use of these tubes has exploded, increasing about 25% *per year* in the 1990s. Recent information reveals that the rate is cresting but conservative estimates are that a quarter of a million elderly people will receive a PEG this year. They are more commonly placed percentagewise in African-Americans and, interestingly, they are more commonly placed if the physician is African-American or Asian. Certain cultural and religious perceptions of food, nutrition, and the right to die inform whether a patient receives a PEG.

There are perverse incentives that might encourage their use as well. Physicians who place them clearly are paid for their services. Endoscopy suites profit as well. Nursing homes derive a double return. Not only do they keep a bed filled by someone who might otherwise possibly die, but both Medicare and Medicaid reimburse the homes more because tube-fed residents purportedly require more staff time. The kicker is that a tube-fed resident actually requires *less* time. A nurse turns the electronic pump on and leaves the room. A resident that is *fed* by mouth calls for staff to sit and feed her.

How does the process unfold that eventuates in a feeding tube? Most commonly, the resident has suffered an acute illness such as a stroke or a severe pneumonia. Alternatively, the resident has reached an advanced or "end" stage of Alzheimer's, Parkinson's, multiple sclerosis, Lou Gehrig's, etc. Staff notices that the resident is no longer capable of feeding herself. When the food is in front of her and presented in an edible form, she cannot use the utensils or her hands properly to move the food to her mouth. When the staff tries to feed the resident, they observe that the resident either coughs or develops a moist sound to her voice. In any event, the food seems to be going down the wrong pipe and that is exactly the case; instead of going into the esophagus leading to the stomach, it proceeds in part down the voice box (larynx) and into the windpipe (trachea). We call this aspiration. Sometimes aspiration is silent, which complicates things even further. Aspiration is problematic because once food and saliva find their way into the lungs, pneumonia (aspiration pneumonia) is the common result.

Why does aspiration occur? The common pathway of a stroke, a serious infection, or advanced Alzheimer's is that each disturbs the normal brain signals that coordinate swallowing. Swallowing is complex and requires split-second timing and the coordination of many groups of muscles. Any disorder of the brain can affect swallowing to the point of aspiration. The dirty little secret is that aspiration occurs even with plain old saliva in the absence of food. The mouth and salivary glands produce upwards of a cup of saliva each day. If swallowing is faulty, a nursing home resident can develop aspiration pneumonia without even eating a speck of food. This explains why feeding tubes do not prevent aspiration pneumonia.

The next team member to become involved is usually the speech therapist. Speech therapists in hospitals and nursing homes have developed expertise in swallowing disorders. Some perform a "bedside swallowing evaluation." In many cases, the patient is made NPO (nothing by mouth) while awaiting the verdict of the therapist. The team often initiates intravenous feeding in order to provide some form of nourishment. The therapist tests the person's swallowing by watching her eat different kinds of food and listening closely for coughing or a change in the quality of her voice. If doubt exists or the therapist wishes to better clarify the swallowing, she will request a modified barium swallow, which is done by the therapist in concert with a radiologist. This is a more sophisticated test in which the food is laced with a material that allows it to be seen by X-ray as it is swallowed. The therapist can also explore a wider variety of foods and techniques but in most cases the bedside test suffices. The therapist might find that swallowing is normal. She might find contrarily that some food proceeds abnormally into the lung. If, significant aspiration or uncoordinated eating occurs, she will test different consistencies of the food and liquid. She may recommend a chopped or pureed diet with or without thickened liquids. The physician at the nursing home or hospital will order this diet and hope for good results. The therapist may, on the other hand, find that any feeding will be risky and recommend an alternate means of nutrition, which is code for a PEG tube.

The juggernaut continues. A nurse sees the recommendations and notifies the doctor, who orders a gastroenterologist to see the patient. The discharge planner is in a hurry to get the patient out of the hospital and pushes everyone for a decision. No one seems able to wait for the tincture of time. In an acute setting, where the ability to swallow can deteriorate quickly due to a sudden illness, it can also begin to recover in a few days, too. Even if the swallowing does not improve, is a PEG tube what the patient would have wanted? Does anyone take a step back to ask about living wills and quality of life?

I have personally only very rarely seen a gastroenterologist talk a family *out* of a PEG tube. I am sure that it happens, but certainly not often. Before you know it, the patient is scheduled and the tube goes in. The unfortunate part is the patient's wishes may have been bypassed completely. The tube does not prevent aspiration pneumonia because that can occur from saliva alone. The tube may not even extend the person's life.

Declining a tube does not mean that you will be starving your loved one. If you choose to avoid a tube, you can still give the staff the go-ahead to feed with caution. If you are working with a reasonable team, the staff spends extra time and takes extra care to feed. Sometimes this is done by spoon, sometimes by a kind of food syringe that looks like a turkey baster. All you are advising (and many homes will have you sign a waiver) is that you *know* there are risks but you are accepting the risks because the quality of life is more important than longevity. None of us lives forever and it is trite but true that *life* is a terminal condition.

A tube also prevents the resident from tasting the food. The ability to taste and enjoy food appears to be important in quality-of-life measures. I wonder how many families who opt for *tubes* consider the paradox that PEG "nutrition" often means never allowing their loved one to taste or enjoy a real meal again. By *declining* the tube and opting for *cautious feeding*, you *will* ensure that your parent gets some personal attention; a human being will be sitting by her side three times a day partaking in one of the oldest of social rituals. I have done my share of feeding residents and it's amazing the kinds of things one talks about, even if it is a one-sided conversation. How can this compare to a nurse entering a lonely room, turning on a machine, and then walking out?

We often assume that PEGs prolong life. Physicians will say things like "you have no choice" or "you can't let your mom starve to death." How I wish I could stick a tube into one of these physicians, tie him up with restraints, deny him the pleasure of tasting food ever again, and consign him to a room without any company while he is "fed."

Another utterance one hears is "let's just try it for a while; you can always take it out." Much like the ventilator, it is very hard, emotionally, to have a tube removed or even to leave the tube in place but shut the feedings off. There are situations when a feeding tube from the outset is a temporary way to boost nutrition to get a patient over the hump and on the road to healing. These are mostly in cases of trauma and major surgery when caloric requirements are much higher than even a young person can consume. When the patient has recovered, the extra calories are not needed. I have removed tubes in these situations and it gives me great pleasure to do so. That's not often the situation in nursing homes.

A cautionary tale: A year ago, a patient was admitted to our home with severe Parkinson's and his second serious bout of pneumonia. He had "failed" his swallowing test and the doctors in the hospital had inserted a PEG feeding tube. His stay with us was stormy and he had several more episodes of pneumonia. For a short while he was able to swallow some food and even walk with assistance, but then he entered a period of steady decline. His wife agreed with a DNR and then a DNH but he somehow managed to stay alive. She finally came to the conclusion that she could not see the man she loved in such a feeble and compromised state. Moreover, she and her three adult children felt that the patient would never have wanted to live like this. She made the brave decision to remove the feeding tube and allow him "to pass" with hospice.

The nurses and aides on the floor and the companion the wife had hired were all distressed that we would be "depriving" him of nutrition. The law was clearly on the wife's side. She was the legal health care proxy. The Supreme Court has ruled, in the Nancy Cruzan case, that artificial nutrition is an extraordinary or heroic measure that need not be given (with the caveat that the individual had made it clear beforehand that he or she would not want to be fed artificially under these circumstances). I sat and talked to the staff and had the director of nursing do the same, but they were having none of it. They didn't come out and disagree publicly, but

I could see from their body language and their huddled conversations that I still needed a leg to stand on. I quickly riffled through the chart and found the living will that the patient himself had filled out years before. It could not have been more specifically, clearly, and convincingly stated that he would not have wanted an artificial tube.

That helped the staff and legally they could not resist. It begged the question, though, of why the doctors had originally inserted the tube. The wife told me she never really wanted it for her husband but the doctors and those close to her had persuaded her to "try it." It all sounded reasonable at the time. Now having made the decision to withdraw the feedings, the wife was beset by guilt. The mind-set of the staff and the verbal and nonverbal messages they sent hurt her. I suspect it will be months to years beyond normal grieving for her to right her ship, if ever. This was a man who had *executed a living will*, for goodness sake, exactly to avoid the situation that ultimately claimed him.

Even if one places a premium on *quantity* over *quality* of life, there is no data that PEG tubes prolong life. The most eloquent writer and thinker on this topic (in my estimation) is my former teacher and colleague, Dr. Muriel Gillick. She is the former physician-in-chief of the Hebrew Rehabilitation Center for Aged, which is the Harvard Medical School's teaching nursing home. She wrote the seminal articles and editorials about tube feedings in the frail and demented elderly. In an article in the *New England Journal of Medicine* she wrote:

> Gastrostomy tubes have not been shown to prolong life, ensure adequate nutrition, or prevent aspiration, and there is neither a secular nor a religious ethical imperative to use them. In addition, they are not necessary to prevent suffering. Since there are

few if any benefits and there is considerable potential for harm, the routine use of gastrostomy tubes in patients with severe dementia is not warranted. Physicians, professional organizations, hospitals, and nursing homes should recommend to patients and their families that nutrition be provided orally, not through a feeding tube, during the final stage of dementia. This approach is distinct from the broader recommendation that patients with advanced dementia receive exclusively palliative care. Decisions about hospice care as opposed to curative care are typically based on an assessment of the quality of life. Decisions about hand feeding versus tube feeding can be made by weighing the pros and cons of gastrostomy tubes.

You go, Dr. Gillick! I do not wish to make light of a serious topic, but until Dr. Gillick began writing, it seemed like gospel that PEG tubes prolonged life. Not only do they not appear to, they can themselves cause medical problems and social isolation. To read more by Dr. Gillick on this issue, you might pick up *Choosing Medical Care in Old Age: What Kind, How Much, When to Stop*. Medical ethicist Dr. Joanne Lynn has also written widely on the topic and her book *Handbook for Mortals: Guidance for People Facing Serious Illness* provides similarly compelling information. If you don't believe me, do your own research. In this most important decision, you should feel satisfied that you have done your homework.

Another useful way to look at the feeding tube has been as a marker of decline and death. The fact that the discussion even arises indicates that the patient is on a trajectory that will soon culminate in death. A useful exercise that we use in the Evercare program is aimed at our nurse practitioners. We want them to address advance directives with their patients when the time is right. We ask them to think about whether they would be surprised if their

patient died within a year. If the answer is yes, then the nurse practitioner needs to discuss end-of-life planning with the patient and/
or the family. This should give you an idea of where your loved
one fits on the spectrum of life and death. If you would not be
surprised that your loved one died within the next year, or if you
have ever stated that your mom has "nine lives," the time is right
to plan. If your mom has been hospitalized several times or had
frequent trips to the ER, the time is right to plan. One could argue
that for anyone about whom you care deeply who has been admitted to a nursing home the time is right to plan.

Substituted Judgment and Final Thoughts

When you do plan, I'd like to leave you with a major principle of
geriatric medical ethics, or for that matter all medical ethics. The
principle is substituted judgment, which means considering what
your mom, dad, uncle, aunt, sister, or brother would want—not
what *you* would want for them or what *you* would want for yourself. When you are looking at your loved one lying in his or her bed,
pretend that she can slip out of bed and stare down at herself in a
lucid state. What do you think she would be saying about the situation? If she could give you advice on what to do or not to do, what
would she say? Many families have told me that this exercise crystal-
lizes for them what advance care planning and substituted judgment
is all about. Let your conscience be your guide, but only if your conscience is conveying what your loved one would be thinking.

I have tried to tell it like it is and I apologize if some of this
was uncomfortable. When choosing a nursing home for your loved
one, *what* you do and *what* you select is most important. When
your loved one is already in a nursing home and has made it her

Communication

Though I pride myself on being a good communicator, especially when it comes to end-of-life care, I have had several times when I missed the mark. In retrospect, I can now see the humor in some of these situations.

- A very ill patient of mine was in the hospital but remained quite lucid and had very good hearing. At some point, the nurses needed to move her to another room and informed the patient's daughter and me. The next time I made rounds, as I was walking out the daughter asked me quietly if I knew when the move would be made. I turned around in her direction and in the direction of the patient and declared, "It's only a matter of time." The next day, my patient seemed forlorn and wouldn't make eye contact. I asked her what the problem was and she said, "It's bad enough to be this sick, but to have my doctor give up on me, too. You said, 'It's only a matter of time'!"

- I took care of a lovely woman years ago in a nursing home in Boston who was not able to make decisions on her own. Her son was her health care proxy. He was an engineer and was very literal. I raised the issue about a DNR for his mom. He asked me very detailed questions and, true to his profession, they mostly concerned numbers and probabilities. He told me he would get back to me. About six months later, his mother none the worse for wear, he left me a message on my voice mail: "Doc, pull the plug."

- The last is perhaps my favorite and points out that what we perceive and what our patients perceive can be two different animals. When I was a resident, our team took care of a sweet-natured elderly woman named Alma who suffered from a hereditary tendency to bleed internally. Forget nine lives, she had *ninety-nine* lives, and at some point every resident in our program had stayed up all night with her during one of her hundreds of admissions to our hospital for severe bleeding. The blood bank frequently worked overtime to match her unusual blood type and provide the numerous pints of blood she received over the years. Finally, my supervising resident, who knew of my budding interest in geriatrics and ethics, asked me to talk to her about advance directives; she had developed several complications and her health was precarious. I entered the room, greeted her, and said, "Alma, if you were to take a turn for the worse and you became gravely ill almost to the point of no return, would you want us to do everything possible to keep you alive?" Highly offended, she answered without missing a beat, "Well, you could at least *try!*"

home, it may be just as important what care you ultimately *don't* select and to what care you *don't* subject her. Less is often more.

Enough of final chapters and end-of-life choices. I hope this guide has been useful in choosing a nursing home and helping your loved one to live well in it. Although I work as a medical director in a nursing home, my most fulfilling days consist of strolling through its corridors as a citizen of the community it represents. I urge you to see yourself not as a visitor but as an integral member of the community, too.

You may be thrilled with the facility and sleep more soundly knowing your loved one is in a warm and caring place. On the other hand, you may have promised your loved one that things would end up differently. As situations arise, be positive and constructive. A major advantage of nursing homes is their small size and the fact that if you handle the situations thoughtfully and treat the staff with respect, most of the time you can effect the changes you want to see. If you stumble, I hope this guide has provided you with resources and ideas to get back up and on track. Become involved with family councils and try to attend meetings about your loved one's care. Visit when you can but also learn to detach yourself when you need to. Use your best judgment and strive for the best, but be aware that better is pretty good, too. Don't be too hard on yourself or expect to return every favor that your relative bestowed on you as a child. On days you cannot scrape together enough time for a visit or a call, still give yourself a pat on the back for trying your best. Being a child of an aging parent is no easy task. By reading this book you are attempting to take care of your loved one as best as you can. If your parent does not or cannot acknowledge this, please allow me to say it: "Thank you."

Index